the "Chief"

the "Chief"

A Biography of
Edward WD Norton, MD

John T Flynn, MD

 TRIAD PUBLISHING COMPANY   GAINESVILLE, FLORIDA

Dut to the events of 9/11/01 and afterward, Library of Congress data was not available at press time. We apologize for any inconvenience this has caused. The following is from our files.
John T. Flynn, 1931–
the "Chief" : A Biography of Edward WD Norton, MD
    by John T Flynn, MD
    ISBN 0-937404-64-0

Published by Triad Publishing Company.
PO Box 13355, Gainesville, FL 32604
www.triadpublishing.com

Nothing that was worthy in the past departs; no truth or goodness realized by this man ever dies or can die; but is still here, and recognized or not, lives and works through endless changes.

—*Thomas Carlyle*

This book is dedicated with admiration and affection to the many, many men and women who, having trained at the Bascom Palmer Eye Institute under Edward Norton, continue the truth and goodness they found there in their own professional lives.

Contents

Preface

IF, AS IGNATIUS OF LOYOLA TELLS US IN HIS SPIRITUAL EXERCISES, character is the will in action, then this is truly illustrated by the life of Edward Walter Dillon Norton, the man who is the subject of this book.

Adversity was his almost constant companion from childhood on, his character forged in the crucible of physical illness that hardened him to life's vicissitudes, yet at the same time left him with a kindness, a softness, a sense of compassion and empathy for the sick for whom he cared. It reached far beyond what is expected of a physician. This man, in the way his life was lived as a physician, was a pure example of the truth of Ignatius' words.

His inner life, while not contradicting anything of that physician's life, revealed, as I have come to know its loneliness and sadness, another dimension that only increases the respect and love I have for him.

His story could well be told simply as a success. A straight line tale of hard work, dedication to an ideal, extraordinary gifts as teacher, physician, planner, leader of professional colleagues, builder of more than an institution, far and away the dominant figure in American Ophthalmology of his day.

All these accolades are his without question. But beyond that is the story of a far more complex individual, unique in his human qualities, simple and unpretentious in his approach to fellow humans, yet subtle and sophisticated in his analysis of their traits, good and bad; kind and compassionate to all who needed it, yet stern and almost biblical in his judgment of those who were dishonest or unethical.

I had the privilege of being associated with Ed Norton for almost three decades of his all-too-short life of 72 years. Did I know him well, or well enough to presume to write this book? Did anyone? For he was an intensely private man who seemed to be always aware of a reality to which we were not privy. And to hold his thoughts well guarded within himself. At best one could only catch glimpses of the workings of his mind when he shared aspects of it with us.

Daily life and what was going on around him clearly fascinated him and he gathered information from everybody he met. He kept to himself his private thoughts and only on the rarest of occasions would he volunteer them and only then when asked. Yet he took in all and saw more clearly the meaning of events for the future as well as the present.

Though he lived within himself, it was never selfishly, always seeming to have time for everybody who needed him. He could and did "walk with kings nor lose the common touch" (Kipling's *If*). His daughter, Carol Ann Rogers, recalled that when she went to pick up his last dry cleaning from the man who cleaned his clothes every week, he said, "I never knew Doctor Norton was so important 'cause he was just such a plain and simple and humble man." Perhaps no words better capture the essence of this extraordinary human.

The strongest reason for my writing this book is to set down on paper, the better to comprehend it, the enormous influence his life had on my life, my career, my goals, in fact the whole shape of my being as a physician. And to share aspects of his life with the many who knew him. In the telling of that life, so full of humor and laughter as well as sadness and pain, glorious accomplishment side by side with tears of loss and grief, we can all come to understand him a little better.

In being around Ed Norton I came to know how beautifully he integrated his own life experience in helping his patients, his colleagues, indeed, anyone with whom he came in contact. But I have only one aspect, one lens through which to view the man. And memory fades and plays tricks on me as time passes. And so I have tried to capture from as many others who knew him, many better than I, how he touched their lives.

If there need be any other reason to write this book it is to describe in words, to recapture, if you will, the wonderful spirit of excellence, of learning and inquiry, the very real joy that came to be known, for those who were part of it, as BPEI. He created it for all of us and it came to be a state of mind, a way of thinking, an art form called the practice of medicine-through-ophthalmology at its highest level. We, who were its fortunate students, carry it with us wherever we go.

If one looks for a definition of the medical profession, one searches in vain in our medical texts. But a paraphrase of the words of the late Supreme Court Justice Lewis Brandeis, a towering legal mind of his generation, in another context, perhaps sums it up best:

> *"Medicine is a profession that is the keeper of a body of knowledge that it advances and passes on to the next generation. It has a code of ethics that includes a component of service to others. The physician places the interest of his patient above self-interest. The profession sets and enforces its own standards and values performance above reward."*

In my almost five decades in medicine, no other institution by its teaching and its culture came closer to exemplifying that definition. It permeated everything we did. And in fulfilling the tenets of that social contact between phyisician and patient that is the essence of our profession, we touch, I believe, the essence of Ed Norton's BPEI.

He created it in the most unlikely of places, Miami, that self-indulgent, hedonistic, suntanned city. He created it in a university, largely unappreciative if not wholly ignorant of the worth of the jewel being built. Created it in a struggling, mediocre medical school riven with nasty, petty political turf battles so characteristic of medical academics.

Indeed, by the time of its opening in 1976, the true essence of what he was about had already begun to slip from his grasp because he had to turn his enormous intellect and focus its formidable powers of concentration on the mundane, almost trivial matters of daily administration. (Not because he wanted to. There was simply no one who could do the job as well as he.) His concerns were to provide each of us—his faculty, his residents, fellows, staff— with the best, most secure working environment possible, always shielding us from its real costs.

Without so much as a word of complaint. Except perhaps to his wife, Mary, and his closest friend and confidant, Victor Curtin. But we will never know, for the one is gone and the other bears a steely reserve on such topics as this, and that Irish reserve is likely to go with him to the grave.

This is so quintessentially an Irish and New England story, built on hard work, endurance, a commitment to excellence through the practice of those virtues, and to a goal almost beyond reach. But I get ahead of myself and my story . . .

On this brilliant, cold Easter Sunday morning, as the ice blue Adirondack sky is caressed by the rose red fingers of the dawn, let us begin the telling.

April 15, 2001
Bolton Landing on Lake George, NY

CHAPTER 1

Where Came He From?

THE STORY OF EDWARD WALTER DILLON NORTON IS IMBEDDED IN the larger story of the toils of the Irish in their own land and the inhospitality imposed on them by an alien power culminating finally in a natural disaster of epic dimension in the middle of the nineteenth century. Deprived of civil, economic and political rights, their religion and language forbidden, and their lands confiscated for the "plantation" of estates from the time of Cromwell, the people lived as little more than serfs and beggars for centuries under the heel of their foreign oppressors in their own country.

And as if nothing worse could befall this hapless race of Celts, famine of monstrous proportions wiped out their potato crop for five years beginning in 1845.

The potato was the staple of the Irish diet. Supplemented by a meager ration of meat, an egg, and few other vegetables, the margin of survival was razor thin. Men, women, infants and children starved by the millions. The famine continued unabated until a lone British politician, out of motives of sheer mercy and humanity, risked his political career by calling on a hostile British Parliament for the repeal of the Corn Laws (designed to protect British agriculture) to allow grain to be imported to the dying satellite isle. That single act of political courage cost Sir Robert Peel his political life but it sustained the life of the surviving Irish people.

They left their native land in waves, until a nation of five million people before the famine dwindled to just over a million at the close of the 1850s. Those who could afford it came in steerage, the hold of the ship, to America. Those without the meager resources to make the trans-Atlantic journey crossed the Irish Sea to England to work in the mines, shipyards and mills during what

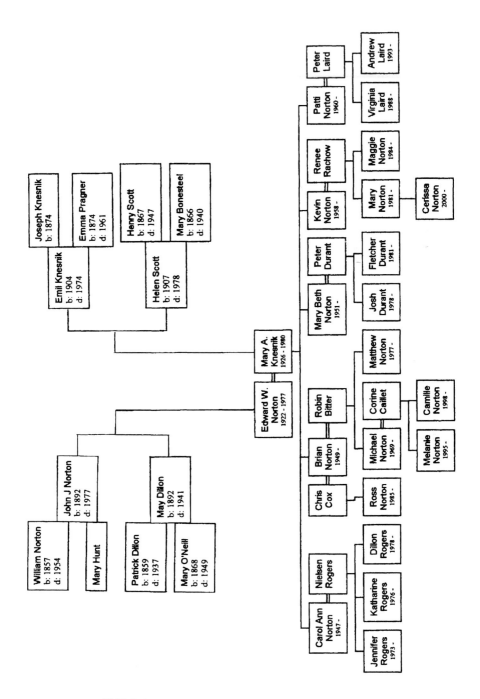

THE FAMILY TREE OF EDWARD W.D. NORTON, MD

was politely known as the Industrial Revolution. They worked side-by-side with English, Scots and Welsh men, women and children, under conditions of human exploitation and privation that beggared description. It was this wrenching social image of human degradation that fueled the fury that found its expression in Karl Marx's *Das Kapital*. And the history of the world for the next century and a half was forever changed.

In this maelstrom of social upheaval, we first pick up the thread of the Norton family tapestry.

William Norton was born in Ballyhaunis, County Mayo, in 1857. He was a bricklayer by trade, an exalted position for an Irishman in the Ireland of that time. He was married to ***Mary Hunt***, who was born in England, in Kidderminster, outside Birmingham. They married in England, and the family immigrated to the United States in the 1880s and settled in Somerville, Massachusetts.

John Joseph Norton, Jack as he was known to family and friends, was born to William and Mary on March 24, 1892, one of six children. He was an avid student and the only one of his family to attend college—Holy Cross, a Jesuit college in Worcester, Massachusetts. An accomplished baseball player, he captained the team and hit the longest home run in Holy Cross baseball history; a plaque to this feat stands today near the center field. For his scholastic and athletic accomplishments he is enshrined in the Holy Cross Hall of Fame.

After graduation Jack played semi-pro ball for a time. But then, as America was inevitably drawn into the "Great War" (as World War I was then known), he enlisted in the US Navy and was trained as a supply officer. During training he attended Princeton graduate school where he was commissioned an ensign in the US Navy in 1918. His service consisted of duty on ships crossing the Atlantic during that war's latter days and after, as this country undertook a huge humanitarian effort to rescue a starving, prostrate Europe from social and political anarchy.

During his college years at "The Cross" Jack met a comely Irish-American girl and after a suitable time of courtship married

May Dillon on July 15, 1919. May was the second of five children: she had three sisters, Margaret, Teresa and Helene, and one brother, John. Though she never went to college, she was extremely intelligent and, along with their father, instilled in her children an early love of learning that persisted throughout their lives.

Jack Norton, son of a bricklayer, became a teacher and later principal of Northeastern Junior High School in Somerville. In 1931 he obtained an AM (Master of Arts) from Boston College, another "blue collar" Jesuit school, in Newton, Massachusetts. He embodied in his life the striving of the immigrant Irish for acceptance and success for which they had so long yearned in their native land. They were destined not to find it there, but in America, slowly and not without travail.

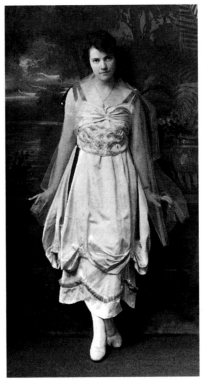

MAY DILLON NORTON

Jack Norton had learned well the virtues of hard work, discipline, and study ingrained in the philosophy of education passed down from Ignatius of Loyola through the Jesuits for four hundred years. His proud and lasting mark in the field of education was that more of his students were accepted to Harvard and other Ivy League schools than from any other public school in the Boston area. Rigorously educated in the classic Jesuit tradition at Holy Cross, he brought that culture with him to Northeastern Junior High School

The Norton family was typical of Irish immigrant America. The father a tradesman or laborer with his hands. The sons moved up the ladder to teacher, civil servant, policeman or fireman. Their sons became doctors, lawyers, architects, politicians, businessmen, clergymen, poets and writers. (A nearby neighbor in Somerville was young Thomas P. [Tip] O'Neill.) For the women, the culture was not yet ready for any role beyond wife, mother and perhaps spinster aunt. Those who worked became the proverbial "Irish working girls": stenographers, telephone operators, department store clerks and waitresses. The forerunners of the working women of today, they embodied the loyalty, devotion to their job, and dependability that made them prized (but never particularly well paid) employees of businesses in the growing, bustling northeastern cities of this country.

May Dillon Norton and Jack Norton were Edward's parents. On their marriage, the couple moved in with her parents, the Dillons, and all three (unmarried) sisters in their home in Somerville. This was very typical of Irish families. Maiden aunts always lived in the home of their parents or a married brother or sister where there was a spare room. There may have been another reason. May's health was said to be none too strong from childhood. Her sisters, in living with them, would be there to be of help, especially when pregnancy, childbirth and children came along.

The forebears of the Dillon family were *Patrick Dillon*, born in 1859 in Roscarberry, Country Cork, and *Mary T. ONeill*, born in Knox, near Clonakilty, County Cork, Ireland. Patrick, a meatpacker, worked at Swift's Meat Packing in Somerville. Eight generations of the Irish branch of the O'Neill family lived in the house where Mary Dillon, Ed's maternal grandmother, was born.

A highlight of a family trip that Ed, Mary, Aunt Teresa and the children took in 1966 is recounted by his daughter Mary Beth: "I remember traveling to Ireland in 1966 and we went to visit the house where Mary (O'Neill) was born. The eighth generation of O'Neills was still living there and my father took pictures of the house and our cousins.

"We just pulled up in our big Thames rental van with all those kids, and my father and Aunt Teresa went in and introduced themselves. The O'Neills were thrilled to meet us. No one (from the family) had ever visited as far as we know. On that trip through Ireland, England and Europe my father was very interested in genealogy, both his and my mother's family."

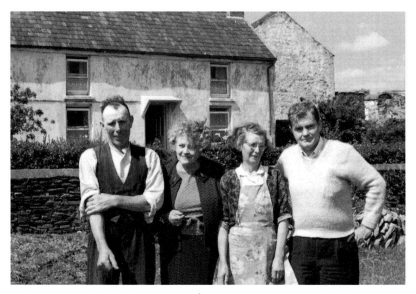

ED NORTON WITH THE O'NEILL FAMILY, IRELAND, 1966

> *This is a refrain that will replay itself again as we describe the man's active mind at play — on vacations and trips throughout his life and throughout the world. Everywhere he found in the simplest of surrounds and with the humblest of people something of interest for his active and engaged mind, ever reaching out to see and hear, to sense the world about him and to understand, better than most, the infinite diversity as well as commonality all humans share.*

We cannot leave this brief sketch of his forebears without recounting a bit of the family background of **Mary Agnes Scott Knesnik Norton**, the love of Ed's life. Mary was the older of two daughters of **Emil Knesnik** and **Helen Gray Scott** of Yonkers, New York. Yonkers was at that time a small town in Westchester county, immediately above the Riverdale section of the Bronx. It stood immediately below a string of towns lining the eastern bank of the Hudson River.

> *These towns, with quaint names such as Hastings-on-Hudson, Dobbs Ferry, Irvington and Tarrytown, figured in the earliest American literature in works of Cooper, Irving and others. Even today they retain a unique charm as the "Hudson River Towns."*

The Knesniks were Czech emigrants from the Austro-Hungarian empire who had immigrated to the US and settled in Yonkers. Emil was the fourth of seven children of **Joseph Knesnik** and **Emma Pragner**. Upon graduation from high school, Emil took a position with his first and only employer, the Peoples Savings Bank of Yonkers, perhaps as a messenger boy. Today the position would probably be disdained as less than even "entry level" and definitely beneath the talents of young job seekers. But through the practice of the simple virtues similar to those of Irish immigrants, Emil rose to become president of the bank.

Emil's wife Helen, born in Yonkers in 1907, was one of four children of *Henry Scott* and *Mary Agnes Bonesteel.* The Bonesteels were early Dutch settlers of New York. Henry Scott was a Scots immigrant, born near Galashiels, in Midlem, Roxburgh, Scotland. He was by trade a painting contractor. Emil and Helen were married as soon as Helen (three years younger than Emil) graduated from high school.

The Knesniks were known in the Norton family as Grandpa and Grandma Knesnik. Their daughter Mary was a graduate of Theodore Roosevelt High School, where she excelled scholastically and socially. The second world war was raging and Mary chose to become part of the war effort by enrolling in the Nurse Cadet Corps at New York Hospital. It is there that she met a young navy V-12 seaman apprentice. But more about that later.

CHAPTER 2

A Sickly Childhood and Sunny Vacations

1922 – 1936

EDWARD DILLON NORTON WAS BORN ON JANUARY 3, 1922 IN the downstairs bedroom at 6 Walter Terrace, Somerville, Massachusetts, the second child of John (Jack) and May Dillon Norton. The house was a large duplex, owned by the Dillon grandparents. Grandmother and Grandfather Dillon and May's sisters lived upstairs and Jack and May and their young family occupied the downstairs. The maiden sisters, in the event anything were to happen to May, would be there to help.

> *May had joined the Navy and was a stenographer at the Boston Navy Yard. At the same time Jack Norton was playing on a US Navy Yard baseball team in Boston. Because regulations forbade marriage between government employees, May was forced to turn in her resignation, which she did on July 14, 1919, the day before her marriage.*

May's health was never robust from childhood. It was said she suffered from rheumatic heart disease, though we have no way of knowing if this were true. Certainly it was the scourge of the children of the northeast during this era.

John Junior (Jackie) was born in 1920, Ed in 1922 and Polly in 1925. Childbearing in those times could be particularly difficult. May had her share and more with all three pregnancies. With Jackie, she had had to go to bed for several months prior to delivery. During that first pregnancy, her husband was away in the US Navy, serving in the supply corps (as he did both during and after the hostilities).

The second infant, Edward, also a difficult pregnancy for May, was known as a "delicate baby." He could not digest regular milk. His parents had to find special milk, known as Walker Gordon (a brand of milk from "certified cows"). It was alleged to be pure, free of any disease and easily digested. Remember, the transmission of tuberculosis via milk was a not-too-distant memory, and pasteurization was not universally practiced then.

Edward attended St. Anne's, a local parochial school in Somerville. He was able to go before the prescribed age because he had learned to read on his own by using his brother Jackie's books. He would read at night and the next morning was full of questions about the meaning of words he had read the previous night.

At age six Edward had his first bout of rheumatic fever, an illness that would dog him throughout his early school years. It was felt at the time to be caused by "chilling" and the effect of cold. Having to kneel on cold concrete to say school prayers was implicated and resulted in his prompt removal from parochial school.

> *The treatment for the condition was absolute bed rest. William Osler's text,* The Principles and Practice of Medicine, *was the bible of those days. It prescribed (in addition to bed rest), salicylates for joint pain, flannel nightgowns, blankets of wool or flannel, no sheets, and a bland diet with lots of milk. Such was the state of medical knowledge of the day by its most eminent practitioner.*

And so, each spring when the rheumatic fever would strike he was removed from school, never finishing a complete year until the eighth grade. The consequences of the illness and its treatment were many. Not the least of which was that the youngster literally was not allowed to take a step, for fear the rheumatic fever would become rheumatic heart disease or glomerulonephritis, its two dreaded consequences. (It was said that during this era Boston's Children's Hospital wards were packed with children with the disease.) Not a step. He had to be carried to the bathroom, eat his meals at his bedside and, most humiliating of all, be brought to the beach in a baby carriage or a stroller.

One can speculate on how this chronic illness and his necessary dependency in early life on others — even when those others were loving parents — helped shape his independence later. He was also silent in later years about anything that affected him physically or mentally.

This silent acceptance of adversity was coupled with a fierce competitive spirit. Although usually kept under tight control, it came out on the tennis court and softball field, and in any occasion of friendly strife, permitting a playful yet fierce competitive fire to reveal itself. As Berchtold Brecht, the Marxist playwright put it, "The will to win is the black curse of the mind." With Norton the will to win was always there but never to win at any price and never to play the game by any but the fairest of rules.

The other side of the coin was his immediate empathy with patients and their illness. It took the form of an uncanny ability to relate to any and all patients without even a word being exchanged.

Because of May's frail health, their family doctor (who was her cousin) advised that they move "to the country." In those years the practice of medicine was largely without a biomedical model of disease. Such remedies as fresh country air and warm climates were part of the few nostrums physicians had available for their sick patients.

It was thus that the family began to summer at Egypt, Massachusetts (post office Scituate), near Cape Cod. The quest for a source of milk for Edward also led the family there because it could be obtained from a nearby farm. The family at first rented a house in summer; later, in 1939, they bought land to a build a home on Hatherly Road for year-round living.

All was not illness and isolation in the life of the Norton family in Egypt. Their house was next to the Cavanaughs and, according to Polly, Ed's sister, they had a wonderful time living by this large family of nine (or was it eleven?) children. Tom Cavanaugh was a fairly well-known figure in the annals of football at Notre Dame.

This may explain Ed's early and deep interest in the for-
tunes of Fighting Irish football, second only to his attachment
to the Boston Braves prior to their departure from Boston for
Milwaukee, and then to the long-suffering and hapless Red Sox.

The water at the beach was too cold for Edward, recovering from rheumatic fever, to learn to swim. Swimming, which became a lifelong joy of his, was learned in the pool at the local YWCA, where the water was warm enough to pose no risk. Up to the age of ten he could go there with his mother and aunts.

Real swimming was reserved for wintertime family visits to South Florida, to a small town called Miami, where Ed perhaps for the first time felt healthy and well. The visits were motivated by

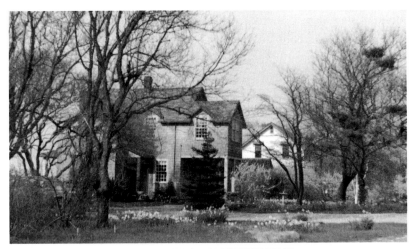

THE HOUSE ON HATHERLY ROAD

Ed's frail health more than any other reason.

The family stayed near the beach. His sister recalls that they would take the bus up Biscayne Blvd. to the beach opposite the Pancoast Hotel (where newlyweds Charles and Ann Morrow Lindbergh were honeymooning). Then take the last bus back in the evening to their hotel. The bus passed the newly built Sears Tower, an art deco building unlike any other Sears in New England. It was an irresistible attraction because the kids could run up and down the wide aisles and could buy live turtles with painted backs for 35¢.

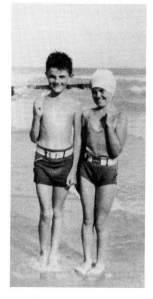

ED AND POLLY IN MIAMI, ABOUT 1930

During this time, Ed began to develop that personal unselfconscious charm that made him so attractive to others. It is said that children with serious illness early in life, on recovery experience a quiet joy quite unknown to their healthy peers. With Edward this took the form of letters to and from his classmates. He had many friends of both genders. So many that Jackie, who had more of a reserved personality than Ed, called his brother's cohort the "League of Nations."

These brief interludes in Miami, with its warm climate and deliciously warm water, were the first imprint of the city destined to play a central role in his life.

As the thirties progressed, May's health waned. The doctor advised them to move to the country full time. Where? Jack and Aunt Theresa scoured the communities around Boston until it became apparent that the house in Egypt, if it could be heated, would do just fine.

By 1939, the family began to occupy the house (a long way from Somerville) year round. At first, May drove Jack (who did not drive) to work in Somerville. That had to stop for reasons of her health, so he learned to drive himself, making the daily commute for many years. The family by then was reduced to three: Jack, May and daughter Polly. The boys were away at Worcester Academy, but more about that later.

Jackie and Ed were close in age and they were also close in their love of sports, particularly baseball. From an early age their father taught them to play the sport from the standpoint of the science of the game as he knew it. Ed continued for years, even into his college days, to play on the Somerville softball team.

In that day, baseball was truly America's national pastime. Ed, along with practically every boy his age, was swept up in its arcana — batting averages of their favorite sluggers, won-lost records of the craftiest pitchers, ERAs, standings versus the hated New York teams that always stood between Boston and the World Series championship they so fiercely coveted and felt they so richly deserved. It consumed the long hours of summer—playing, reading about it, talking and arguing about it, living the slow drama that unfolded day by day throughout the 154-game season until it was time for the World Series and back to school after Labor Day.

Eventually Edward decided, since he was not talented enough in the sport to play professionally in the big leagues (would his goal ever be anything less?), he would be the "announcer." The early pioneers of the radio became heroes in their own right to the games' true devotees. He practiced assiduously in the summer afternoons miming the voice and phraseology and dialogue of Fred Hoyle, the Braves' radio announcer.

And at his confirmation, the sacrament in which the baptized member of the Catholic faith affirms commitment to that faith, he took as his saint's name (part of the sacramental rite), Walter, after Saint Walter—but also Walter Berger, his favorite player on the Boston team. And so he became Edward Walter Dillon Norton . . . or EWDN, the Chief, as we came to know him later.

CHAPTER 3

Worcester Academy and Harvard

1937 – 1943

THE NORTON BOYS, JACKIE AND ED, WERE NOW TEENAGERS. THOUGH they had become members of that particular age, it probably had no cult-like significance as it now has in this country. The times were far too serious for such trivia.

The entire developed world was trapped in a severe depression, unlike anything seen before in the twentieth, indeed in any century. Men, out of work by the millions, took to wandering the dusty roads as homeless drifters looking for work, any work to give them back a morsel of self-respect and money to buy food to slake the hunger gnawing at the bellies of their children. Whole families were hungry, even to the point of starvation

Abroad, there was widespread loss of faith in a capitalist system that seemed unable to right itself, put people back to work, and address the needs of a dispirited, quietly angry and alienated populace. Franklin Roosevelt became president, and while the efforts of his government, subsumed under the title of the New Deal, had given the people hope in 1933, by 1935–36 much of that had been dissipated. In Europe and Asia, totalitarian dictatorships, bent on world hegemony and led by ruthless, iron-willed men, were rising from the near total wreckage of formerly productive economies.

These brutal police states that crushed all rights and dissent seemed to many to address the more basic needs of desperate, hungry and unemployed people. They would play a critical role in the history of the rest of the century as it unfolded. It was a very dangerous and serious time in the history of the world.

Though privation was not a threat in the Norton home, a certain seriousness of purpose, reinforced by world events, was. Jack Norton's position in the public school system was unthreatened by the layoffs that hovered over the shoulder of many men his age. At first as teacher, then principal of Northeastern Junior High, he had established a culture of learning, emphasizing the classics. Everyone took Latin. Everyone studied in the classic mode of the Jesuits as Jack had learned at "the Cross." Hard work, discipline, study and attention to detail—serious application of the dedicated mind was the *leitmotif* of this tradition.

Its prize was success for those who made the effort, and the Norton boys surely did. Both excelled at Somerville High School and later Worcester Academy where they transferred for their last two years before college. They maintained contact with the family in the time honored way that males have always maintained contact with their homes when they leave for school. Weekly came a brown paper package tied up neatly with string, containing their laundry. There were also occasional phone calls and a letter or two.

It came time to think of college. May wanted Jackie to go to Williams College, which she considered a better academic institution than Harvard. At least for Jackie. It was small, with small classes and a reputation for close faculty-student interaction. It provided the kind of atmosphere she knew he needed, for he was more shy and socially reserved than Ed.

May, though never a college graduate herself, was a keen observer of human nature and how higher education could shape that nature. Money, however, made the decision, and the family, with three children to educate, chose the less expensive Harvard; tuition at the time was about $400 per year.

The family looked upon Harvard in a far less flattering light than it is held today. Harvard accepted the playboy sons of its wealthy graduates, demanding little effort from them. It was cold and impersonal, its famed faculty far distant from the students who came to learn and worship at their feet.

Not everyone agreed that this was the opportune time for Ed to go to Harvard. He was only seventeen when he applied. But the Norton boys came with the virtues instilled by their father, honed by solid accomplishments in a good preparatory school; Harvard might just provide a good education. But George M. Hosmer, head of the college preparatory course at Worcester Academy, did not believe that Ed was ready for Harvard because of his youth and shy nature.

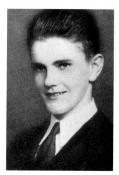

*EDWN COLLEGE
APPLICATION PHOTO*

General Estimate

The Committee on Admission will be very grateful for an estimate of the candidate's character. They will be glad to have information about the candidate's scholarly interests, whether connected with his school work or outside of it; his possession of exceptional ability of any kind, his fondness for outdoor sports, his manly qualities, such as truthfulness, courage, generosity, and regard for duty; the moral influence he has exerted among his schoolmates, and any ways in which it has been recognized. The Committee do not expect, of course, that information will be given on all the points mentioned above. Whatever information is received will be placed on file in the office of the Committee, and will be accessible to administrative officers only.

        Edward Norton is a brother of John Norton, a member of the present freshman class at Harvard. Edward is a quiet, rather shy boy. He undoubtedly is a persistent worker, and does his best at all times. I seriously doubt, however, the wisdom of his attempting Harvard next year. He is young and immature. As I have seen his work in my English class, and as the instructor in French has seen it, he seems lacking in the speed and power that he will need in college. Our judgment appears confirmed by his Otis score and also by his deficiency in vocabulary. He might succeed in college, but I feel strongly that he should have another year of training and maturity to make him safe. He is a youngster of fine qualities.

HOSMER'S EVALUATION OF EWDN

Even so, Ed was admitted to Harvard College in September, 1939. Hosmer's words seemed prophetic; Ed struggled academically in his first two years and was put on probation. But by his junior year his record improved dramatically, to the level of distinction. He was showing a distinct aptitude for mathematics and the sciences; his mind opened to their innate rigor and consistency.

This experience was something Ed took with him into later life; he always placed more value on the student who started off slowly (perhaps with difficulty) but later improved and finished on an upward course, than the student who did academically well from the outset.

March 4, 1940

Dear Mr. Norton,

I am glad to inform you that the Administrative Board has voted to take no action at present in regard to your record, other than permitting you to continue on probation. As you realize, your mid-year record of three courses is insufficient for the promotion requirements.

Should you experience any difficulty in carrying five courses this term I wish you would let me know. I trust you will not hesitate to come in at any time for a discussion of your work.

Sincerely yours,

KNIGHT W. McMAHAN

Mr. E. W. D. Norton
MacPherson Avenue
Scituate, Massachusetts

LETTER TO ED NORTON RE PROBATION AT HARVARD

Ed was a day student at Harvard. Day students at that time were for a variety of reasons not part of the campus life culture. Many lived nearby with relatives and it saved a considerable expense to do so. (Ed lived with Grandmother Dillon and the aunts in Somerville.) Many had to work to pay the tuition and went from the classroom to the factory floor. Some were married and lived at home with their wives.

All were isolated socially from campus life. They had their own social structure, about which we know little. Their gathering place on campus was Claverly Hall, where they ate their midday meal. What little participation they had in campus life took place there. Not really social outcasts, they were a separate and probably just a little bit unequal stratum of Harvard life.

Ed's daughter Mary Beth accompanied her father to his 50th class reunion in 1993. She recalls quite vividly his pleasure in meeting many of his classmates of that year's vintage for the first time.

But Edward Norton, the student, had had little time for the carefree frivolities of campus life. Events within the family and on the world stage were closing in.

His mother's health, always suspect, worsened in 1941. According to one account (that could not be verified), she developed a streptococcal infection for which she was given a sulfa drug. Her physician was unaware of the damaging effect that the early sulfa drugs could have on the kidneys of some patients with already impaired function. In spite of frantic efforts by all to save her, she died on June 29, 1941, within five days of being given the drug. In their grief the family felt her death was due to the physician's ignorance.

May's death was a family tragedy, not because she was healthy (quite the contrary, her health had always been a concern to all even before her marriage), but because she played such a vital role in the family. Now she was gone.

Jackie, Ed's brother was inconsolable. His reaction to his mother's death as well to what was happening in the world led to his early departure from Harvard and enlistment in the United States army as a private. This caused much consternation in the family, as the life expectancy of enlisted men, especially privates, was not very high, especially as the country was engaged immediately in a two-front war against formidable and well-prepared opponents.

He rebuffed all family entreaties to at least apply for Officer Candidate School. "If they want me they'll find me" was his *sang froid* response. And find him they did. As a commissioned officer in the combat engineers, he saw action in North Africa and Europe throughout the second world war.

After the war he did not return to Harvard but completed his education in engineering at Syracuse University. After graduation he worked as a civil engineer. He never spoke of his wartime experiences with his nieces and nephews.

We know little of Jack Norton's grief. Their marriage was of only twenty-one years' duration. In 1944 Jack married May's sister Helene, and the two families, Norton and Dillon, became even closer. Helene was always known to later generations of Nortons as Aunt Helene.

Ed was obviously bonded to his mother by shared illness and the special caring that members of a family have for one another who know that burden. But on another level Ed was closer to her in his keen interest in and perception of everything in his world, as she was in hers. They were kindred spirits, I believe.

Ed, who was nineteen in December 1941, chose a different path to assuage his grief. He remained at Harvard, continued his education, and worked in the Boston office of the FBI on the 12 to 8 AM "graveyard shift," to provide money for his Harvard tuition and savings for his contemplated medical education.

This era had about it a highly charged ambience. Boston was an Atlantic seaboard city that could at any time come within gun range of prowling German Raiders, U-boats or saboteurs. It was under stringent blackout conditions in an atmosphere of tightened security.

One night in November, 1942, when Ed was on duty, a fire destroyed the Cocoanut Grove nightclub, taking 492 lives and resulting in hundreds of burned and severely injured patients.

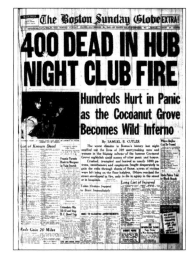

Although simply a clerk on the night shift, Ed remained at his post for over ninety hours. It was during this awful event and its aftermath that he was recognized by co-workers as a "future J. Edgar Hoover" (which at the time was the highest compliment that could be paid an FBI employee by his colleagues) if he had chosen this path.

The director of the Boston FBI office wrote a letter of recomendation to the admissions committee of Cornell, in which he singles out Ed for his exceptional devotion not only to his regular duties but to others he assumed when necessary.

Ed's dedication to the task at hand displayed as well another of his singular virtues, for which he later became justly famous: his lack of need for sleep.

Ed's record at Harvard continued to improve in impressive fashion in his third and final year. It firmed his decision on medicine as his career. Considering his own medical history, and his mother's, this was not an inappropriate choice.

After applying to Harvard Medical School, he was granted an interview but was not accepted. There was probably a congerie of many reasons. His early difficulties with course load? His night work at the FBI, which probably detracted from study time? (But he worked there during his years of success as well.) An admission policy that favored the sons of Harvard grads? We'll never know.

He dealt with it as one would expect him to deal with life's disappointments. "If you can meet with triumph and disaster and treat those two imposters just the same . . ." (*If,* Kipling again). After carefully surveying a number of the available schools, he chose Cornell Medical College, New York Hospital.

Edward W. D. Norton received his Baccalaureate degree from Harvard College on March 1, 1943, as the war in Europe and Asia reached a crescendo of violence and human slaughter, of horror unparalleled in human history.

CHAPTER 4

Cornell Medical School

1943 – 1946

IN JULY, 1943, EDWARD WALTER DILLON NORTON, AGE TWENTY-one, entered the freshman class of Cornell Medical College, New York Hospital, one of a class of eighty-eight.

> *A colleague described him as "a short but rather handsome guy with lots of black hair and a winning smile," a description that fit him well for most of his life.*

He was assigned living quarters (a room on the fifth floor in the old nurses residence) on York Avenue between 69th and 70th Streets, just north of the school and next to the new nurses residence. The quarters were spartan; each small room had a desk, a sink and a bed.

In every sense the education system had a heavy military overtone. During these wartime years, all students at medical schools, if physically and mentally fit, were automatically enrolled in an armed service education program and on an accelerated course of learning. Doctors were turned out in three rather than four years. They went to class year-round, dressed in the service uniform of their branch.

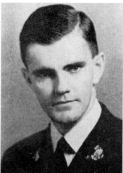

ED NORTON, 1944

Ed was no exception; apparently his childhood rheumatic fever had left no permanent damage. At the end of the freshman year he was inducted into the Navy V-12 program as a seaman apprentice. He wore the uniform of a seaman apprentice with an anchor as insignia, much as did trainees elsewhere (save Annapolis). He and his classmates had to report for roll call and drill at 6:30 AM.

Everyone was impressed with how serious a student Ed was. Indeed, his notes were painstaking in their accuracy. They were note-worthy in another respect. Mature beyond his years of medical education, Ed always reached beyond the simple rote copying that passes for so much medical education (particularly in its first two years) to make the clinical connections.

His interests were already pointing in the direction of the visual and central nervous systems. Particularly pertinent is his description in his third year notebook of bulbar palsy, an entity he would soon experience first hand. Ed's hard work and probing intelligence were rewarded with induction into AOA (Alpha Omega Alpha, medical student honor fraternity) in his senior year.

This was the golden era of New York medicine, and education at Cornell proved a wise choice. Russell L. Cecil, MD, was Professor and Chair at Columbia-Presbyterian and Robert F. Loeb, MD, held the same position at Cornell-New York Hospital. Their *Text-*

CLINICAL DESCRIPTION OF BULBAR PALSY, 1945

NOTES, NEUROLOGY OF THE BRAINSTEM, 1945

book of Medicine had replaced Osler's as the bible for medical students, and their faculties boasted a surfeit of the brightest minds of the day.

Among that group of dynamic and charismatic teachers were Bronson Ray, the neurosurgeon and last student of Harvey Cushing at Harvard, and Harold Wolff, the neurologist. It goes without saying that these two men dominated their respective specialties in New York medicine and perhaps the entire country.

Although always an admirer of Bronson Ray (and the admiration became mutual for it was said that he would perform a craniotomy on a patient solely on the basis of an Ed Norton field), it was Harold Wolff to whom Norton was drawn. Wolff was an inspiring man with a great intellect and a vast interest in and command of his subject; as a teacher he was unsurpassed. He touched his students' minds in a very deep way.

In Ed's sophomore year, Thomas Hedges, a freshman from Cleveland, Ohio, moved in next door to him. The two became close friends throughout medical school and their later careers in ophthalmology, which were to mirror each other in many respects.

Ed and Tom, despairing of ever learning neuroanatomy from the textbook's two-dimensional drawings and the glass slides posted weekly on the windows of Professor George Papanicolaou's histology laboratory, spent countless hours in the laboratory of the Payne Whitney Psychiatric Clinic building a clay and wire model of the brain in three dimensions. It was this exercise that formed the earliest basis for Ed's uncanny and intimate knowledge of the structure of the brain and its connections, which stayed with him throughout his life. Neurology as a specialty seemed to loom large in the minds of both men.

But as so often happens to medical students, when the next specialty area opens its store of hard won clinical wisdom to their hungry, developing minds, they quickly desert their commitment to yesterday's service for the rapture of today's. Such is the process. And it's not due to any fickleness of their nature but rather to the wonder of the human body's infinite, varied and fascinating mysteries. And above all to a mentor, a teacher, a role model.

Bronson Ray and Harold Wolff were Ed's first mentors. Then the third striking teacher of that talented group appeared, to add his luster to the emerging shape of Norton's career. John Milton McLean in 1942—shortly after the end of his chief residency and a year's faculty appointment at the Wilmer Institute of Ophthalmology of Johns Hopkins University—barely thirty-two, assumed the post of Professor and Chief of the division of Ophthalmology at Cornell.

For the youngest professor of ophthalmology in the United States to step into that position was a tribute to his awesome brilliance. John McLean was the acknowledged leader during his training; "the Prince," as he was known to the group of Hopkins residents who trained with him. With names such as Maumenee and Guyton, it may have been the best crop of residents ever to come from that institution.

All three men, Ray, Wolff and McLean, very different in personalities and demeaner, but dedicated and inspired teachers, had a profound influence on Ed Norton.

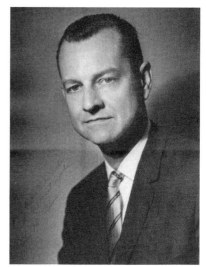

JOHN MC LEAN, MD

If the word-pictures I have drawn of him make my subject sound a bit one-dimensional, nothing could be farther from the reality. Ed was at all times as fun loving as only an Irishman can be. He was a serious student and had his priorities right but he could enjoy a good laugh, a good party, a good story, a good joke, a good song (sung hideously off key) — all that and more, but only when the work was all done.

Although Ed's studies always came first, on occasion he found time to join his classmates at Tom's Tavern on First Avenue for a round or two.

Edward Dunlap, a lifetime friend as well as teacher, has among his earliest recollections of Ed Norton, a vague memory of seeing him on a Saturday afternoon for a racketball injury to one of his eyes—fortunately not a severe one. Safety glasses were probably not much in style in those days.

In January 1945, as a junior, Ed met a vivacious, outgoing, joyful young cadet student nurse, Mary Knesnik. She was extraordinarily popular. According to her daughter, Carol Ann, Mary had joined the corps of nurse cadets training at New York Hospital because a number of her high school friends were early casualties in the war.

> *It was an infectious public-spirited ethic and its hold on the young was especially strong. Literally everybody wanted to be part of it. It was probably the last time this country was gripped with such fervor and felt so genuinely good about itself and where it was going. The war had brought an end to the depression as well as giving us a sense of purpose.*

One day in February, 1945, Mary Knesnik (in her own words) "saw a young man writing copious chart notes on Neurology, G-2 floor. I had never seen him before and now saw him only from the back . . . my maternal feelings (or something) were aroused by this short (5' 8½"), slim teenage-looking boy (he was 22) and I went over and rumpled his hair. He looked up, rather bewildered, with his young Irish face and green eyes . . . I introduced myself and asked his name. It was Edward Walter Dillon Norton. A friend told me later that he had been trying to work up courage to ask me to a fraternity beer-party dance . . . we courted on East River Drive (pedestrian walk), Central Park Zoo, the museums . . . anything free, because he was a poor boy and was buying war bonds."

The twenty-three-year-old midshipman doctor-in-training and

the cadet nurse were engaged that July and married in December. Anybody could see years later from the warmth and joy that radiated from both that they were a ying and yang pair.

Mary resigned from her student nurse status (possibly because of the same regulation that in 1919 stymied May Dillon from marrying Jack Norton and remaining in government service) and married Edward Norton on December 15, 1945, at Saint Joseph's Church in Bronxville, New York, near the Knesnik home.

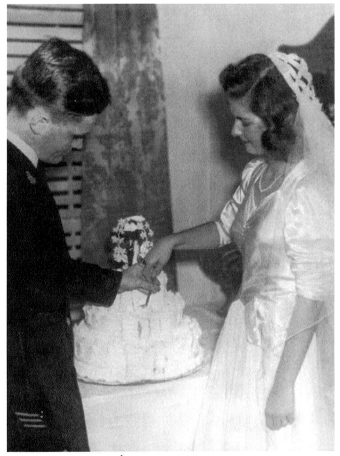

ED AND MARY'S WEDDING, DECEMBER 15, 1945

Bronxville at the time was known as the "Irish" suburb among the many posh such settlements in Westchester County. It had earned the sobriquet because it numbered among its inhabitants a healthy minority of the sons and daughters of Irish immigrants. Parishioners at St. Joseph's included Joe and Rose Kennedy and their brood, and their son Ted was married there.

The Nortons had their wedding reception at the Knesnik home and they honeymooned for three days at Aunt Evie's (Knesnik) place in Ridgefield, Connecticut. Evie kept live chickens and, according to family lore, left one for the newlyweds to dine on. The task of killing it was left to Ed, being the male. But he possessed no more skills in this art than most males, and ended up with a decapitated chicken running around the yard spurting blood in the snow, much to the amusement of his bride. Evie was kind in another way as well; she equipped their marriage bed with cow bells and similar romantic paraphernalia.

A very special bond was formed between Ed and Mary so strong that it enabled them to embrace as part of their family, not only their five children but many, many surrogate children that they met along life's way and somehow make them all feel part of that family.

And so ended an eventful three years at Cornell for Edward Walter Dillon Norton. He was graduated March 31, 1946, and on graduation was commissioned a Lieutenant (junior grade) in the US Navy. He was soon to be placed on detached duty, to intern at Cincinnati General Hospital. In somewhat less than clear focus were the main sheet anchors of his future profession, involving the visual system as the paradigmatic example of the nervous system; he would study under men who were among its most effective and notable teachers.

CHAPTER 5

Cincinnati General and on to the US Navy

1946 – 1949

LET US SET THE SCENE AS IT MIGHT HAVE APPEARED TO A YOUNG doctor on his way to an internship at Cincinnati General Hospital in 1946.

This was a coveted internship for many reasons. It had one of the country's best full-time faculties and had already adopted the model of salaried physicians whose primary role was not developing a large private practice, but rather developing a practice as a tertiary referral center to see the most complicated and demanding types of medical problems. Teaching from these patients who sought their professional care was their *metier*. It may well be that this was his first exposure to what he brought to a high state of perfection in his own department in later years.

> *The community doted on their hospital as did the Procter and Gamble company, the town's leading employer. The Procter family still played a large role in the management of the business, and William Procter, the childless last member of the family, willed his entire fortune to the Children's Hospital of Cincinnati, instantly making it the wealthiest endowed children's hospital in the United States if not the world.*

The city, rather old-fashioned in its mores and heavily Germanic and hardworking in its ethos, was situated on the northern bank of the Ohio River. Directly across was Covington, Kentucky, where loose morals, gambling and all kinds of ribald fun was to be had; this was frowned upon by the good burghers, though on occasion one or other of them was known to sneak across the river to witness, at least, the loose and lively lifestyle of those lost souls.

Both cities were surrounded by seven hills, likened by the natives to the Seven Hills of Rome. This truly was heartland America, a perhaps slower paced and considerably less noisy world than what Ed and Mary knew on 68th Street and York Avenue on the east side of Manhattan Island.

What were the times in which they lived? World War II was ended and supposedly America was at peace. The huge standing army and navy the country had raised by conscription, twelve million in number, was in the process of headlong demobilization. It was an armed force composed almost entirely of drafted civilians with a thin cadre of regular army and navy to lead it.

The war over, they (the civilians, that is) wanted out of the military in the worst way. But as Abraham Lincoln had said prophetically to his countrymen on another critical occasion in the life of this country (his last State of the Union address delivered in March of 1865), barely a month before his assassination, "We must think anew, we must act anew, the dogmas of the quiet past are insufficient for the troubles of today.; we cannot escape history."

And neither could these United States as a country escape history in 1947. On the horizon and in the counsels of government were the first worried glances cast eastward at the stirrings of a potentially expansionist Soviet Union. Northern Iran had been occupied under a pretext of restoring order and suppressing banditry. Greece was torn by civil war between the *ELAS,* a communist dominated resistance movement that alone had fought a bloody guerrilla war against the occupying Nazi armies, and the loyalists and monarchists who, though the legitimate government prior to the war, had fled Greece with the approach of the *Wehrmacht* but returned to claim the right to resume that legitimacy after the war.

Western Europe itself was prostrate, its economies wrecked, its industrial plant and transportation system laid waste by aerial bombardment. Most importantly, its people were demoralized and guilt stricken by the black stain of collaboration and even support for Adolph Hitler and his ruthless and brutal destruction of innocent people by the millions, now revealed for all the world to see in merciless, flickering black-and-white images of the newsreel films.

Europe was starving, its once proud civilization shorn of its dignity and humanity by images of concentration camps and its collaborators' trials. Communist parties were strong and noisy in western Europe and threatened to take over power democratically at the polls. And just might have but for clandestine financial support with US dollars funneled to opposition parties by the CIA.

The so-called "cold war" had not yet been so declared by that sly, silver-tongued English politician, Winston Churchill. A largely unknown and untested president, Harry Truman, now occupied the White House that had been home to Franklin Roosevelt and his family for twelve years. It seemed to many that this simple, plain-spoken midwesterner, a product of one of the last surviving urban democratic political machines, could never replace the steady hand and patrician voice that had steered the country's destiny for longer than any man in history.

But steer it he must, and a crucial aspect of that was to keep the framework of an armed force intact, particularly its officer corps and support services, should it be needed. An unpopular move politically but he took the heat for it, just as he was to do for many decisions during his eventful terms in office.

Since July 1945, in his hands alone rested a new and awesome weapon, the atomic bomb, which was to menace the human race with extinction. History was frozen by these awful events: WWII and its aftermath, and the bomb for the rest of the twentieth century. There was little chance that this country would be able to escape history in these trying times.

And so the young naval officer-physician was not discharged, but detached for temporary duty as an intern at the civilian hospital of his choice. He selected and was accepted at Cincinnati General Hospital. The internship was for fourteen months, and presumably (we have few records) he rotated through medicine, surgery, ob-gyn, pediatrics, in- and outpatients and the subspecialties.

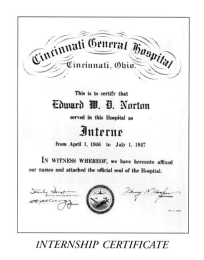

INTERNSHIP CERTIFICATE

Far more important for the young marrieds was the fact that Mary became pregnant with their first child and was due to deliver at almost precisely the same time that Ed was called back on active duty. Ed was ordered to the Oakland Naval Hospital to await further orders. Mary returned to Yonkers to be with her parents (the Knesniks) for the birth, and waited for word to join Ed for what was presumed to be service at a west coast military hospital.

Carol Ann was born at New York Hospital on August 17, 1947, a lovely, healthy infant. As a grown woman and a mother herself, Carol Ann recalls that Mary told her that people who knew Ed at New York Hospital would come in and say, "Oh she looks exactly like her father." And there is some truth in that, as the Norton children all share a strong resemblance to Ed, blended and softened by the feminine features of their mother. Ed, because of service obligations could not be there, but mother and child were surrounded by doting grandparents, sister and friends of the couple from earlier NY Hospital days.

A bombshell arrived shortly thereafter in the form of a telephone call from Ed to Mary. Ed had orders to join a ship stationed in Japan, for active duty. It was far from the outcome they expected. To Mary, it meant her husband would be leaving for an overseas assignment in a war-desolated land, far from home, for who knew how long? What was she to do?

This dilemma is recalled by Carol Ann: "I remember my grandmother talking about how upset my mother was, and in tears . . . because she would have to stay behind and that he wasn't going to be able to see either of us."

This was not an isolated event, nor did it single out the Nortons. The world was undergoing rapid realignment of its power relationships. Out on its farthest perimeter was where the soulless game of Realpolitik was being played out by the surviving powers of the second world war, the Soviet Union and the United States. The British Empire, severely wounded due to its heavy manpower losses in the first (so-called "great") war, caused largely by the stupidity and incompetence of its class-ridden general staff, was bankrupt and drained after this second war. So were other traditional imperial and colonial powers: France, Italy, Belgium.

Into the power vacuum swiftly moved the totalitarian dictatorship of Joseph Stalin in the Soviet Union. Our ally during World War II, it now appeared, if not yet an enemy, vaguely menacing and unfriendly. On the sacrifice and blood of Russian civilians and armies, the Russian people had broken the back of the German Wehrmacht in a mortal struggle not for the survival of Marxian versus National Socialist ideology but for the survival of Mother Russia, absorbing tremendous casualties numbering more than all the rest of the combatants of the war combined. As a consequence, the Soviet empire stretched from the Elbe River in divided Germany to the Kurile Islands in the Sea of Japan.

At the other pole of this power struggle stood the United States, alone among the victorious combatants of the war with its economy intact and its people largely unscarred. Its armed forces, made up largely of civilians who, once the conflict was over, resumed a healthy disregard for the regimentation and authoritarianism inherent in the nature of military services.

The self-effacing midwesterner in the White House faced this state of affairs with a sense of equanimity for which he received little credit. He rose to the challenge wherever it arose and brought his fellow citizens, often grumbling and complaining about his shortcomings, to assume their role inherent in the bipolar world of democracy, with all its drawbacks, versus the ideology of state communism. And with this radical realignment, the major outlines of the post-war world for the next half-century began to emerge.

The United States, a third-class military power prior to the war (19th behind those two perennial South American superpowers and enemies, Paraguay and Uruguay), would, in its aftermath, become a colossal military power for the rest of the century.

The darkened clouds lifted somewhat and the fates smiled on the young couple, though briefly. In its infinite wisdom the Navy's "BuPers," or more properly the Bureau of Personnel (the real beginning of the alphabetical dumbing down of the English language that I believe originated in the USN), did not know the whereabouts of the ships of the huge two-ocean Navy. That was the province of "BuShips."

It had made a small mistake: it had misplaced the whereabouts of the ships to which Ed, the Lieutenant (jg)-doctor had been assigned. The ships in question were a squadron of four destroyers belonging to "Desdiv" (Destroyer Division), 32-itself consisting of a complement four squadrons.

His squadron's ships were home-ported in San Diego as was one other squadron, and not in Japan where the other two squadrons were on station. Had he flown to Japan under the misapprehension of its whereabouts, he would, of course, have immediately been issued orders to another billet in Japan for the duration of his enlistment.

The gods smiled and the family crisis melted. Mary and her infant daughter Carol Ann made the transcontinental journey and joined Ed in what was at the time standard issue base housing quarters for newly commissioned officers, rooms in a quonset hut.

There is no better summary of his shipboard service than the letter (probably, at the time, squadrons were under the command of a full commander; only later did it become a Captain's billet), from Commander R.R. Conner, his commanding officer, to Harold Wolff, MD, the neurologist under whom Ed studied on his return to civilian life and Cornell.

Another crisis of potentially devastating impact soon arose to beset the young couple. Homer F. Schroeder, MD (known to all as Fritz), a friend and fellow draftee-physician stationed at Oakland Naval Hospital, went to visit Ed and Mary over the Labor Day weekend in September, 1948. Thinking to find Ed aboard ship, he was told that the young medical officer went home because of a cold and a sore throat.

Fritz made his way to the quonset where the family was living and met Mary, pregnant with Brian, their second child. Ed was sacked out and Fritz decided to stay the night in the quarters next door, which happened to be vacant.

EXECUTIVE OFFICER
RECEIVING STATION, SAN DIEGO
U.S. NAVAL REPAIR BASE
SAN DIEGO 36, CALIFORNIA

February 4, 1949.

Dr. Harold Wolff,
Veterans Administration Hospital,
130 West Kingsbridge Road,
Bronx 63, New York.

Dear Doctor:

Lieutenant (junior grade) E. W. D. Norton, Medical Corps, USNR, asked me if I would write to you in connection with his application for Residency Training in your Hospital.

I was fortunate in having Doctor Norton serve in my command as Division Medical Officer during the period of about one year, while I was Division Commander of Destroyer Division THIRTY-TWO. As Division Medical Officer, he was responsible for the Medical Department of four Destroyers, each with a complement of 270 men. Doctor Norton often remained aboard ship after hours in order to administer to his patients and voluntarily called on families of Navy personnel ashore in order to be of service. He successfully organized and supervised athletic teams which greatly improved morale. He appeared at all times keenly interested in his medical profession and at the same time mindful of his duties as a Naval officer.

I can frankly say that during my twenty-three years in the Naval Service I have never been associated with a more capable, conscientious, loyal, and general all around superior young medical officer. He is a young man of high ideals and a very pleasing personality that invites confidence.

I consider the medical profession privileged to be represented by Doctor Norton, and I sincerely feel that any consideration that may be accorded him will greatly benefit the profession. If I may answer any questions you might have or in any way assist Doctor Norton in obtaining a Residency, I will be very happy to do so.

Respectfully,

R. R. Conner

RRC:gs

LETTER TO HAROLD WOLFF FROM COMMANDER CONNER

In the early morning hours of the next day, Ed woke Fritz up and said, "Hey Doc, I think I've got polio, my uvula is paralyzed." He later told Carol Ann that he had gotten up during the night to get an aspirin and a drink of water, and when he tried to swallow, he couldn't, and he regurgitated the water through his nose. For a man with his clinical acumen the diagnosis was easy: bulbar polio, the most dreadful form of the disease.

They drove to the hospital where Ed was seen by a Dr. Evans, Chief of Medicine at the Naval Hospital, who felt Ed did not have polio but ordered a spinal tap to be sure. In Fritz's words, "Old Ed was right. He did have bulbar polio."

> *The 1948 epidemic was particularly virulent from the standpoint of the tissue attacked by the virus. The brainstem, as opposed to the spinal cord, was its hallmark. Iron lungs were set up in armories across America because hospital beds were filled to capacity.*

Ed Norton was one of only two survivors of bulbar polio that year in San Diego. He was hospitalized, put in Trendelenberg position on blocks because he couldn't handle his saliva. He did not require an iron lung. Fritz stayed with him at the doorway of his room and kept him up on the news of Mary and Carol Ann, both of whom were quarantined in their quarters in the quonset hut.

It was through this experience that Fritz became very close to the Norton family. After both men were discharged from the service and pursuing post-graduate training, Ed in ophthalmology in New York and Fritz in obstetrics-gynecology in Philadelphia, that Fritz met Mary's little sister Janet, and the rest, as they say . . . but that's another story.

Regarding his assessment of his friend (and brother-in-law), Fritz had this to say, "I must say that Ed is the smartest doctor I ever met, perhaps the smartest individual I ever met."

Sea duty with a destroyer squadron was out of the question for the convalescent. While still a recovering in-patient he got himself assigned duty on Dr. Meyer Weiner's ophthalmology service. By then he had made his choice. By what road he arrived at this choice

U.S. Naval Hospital
San Diego, California
December 8, 1948

Dr. Harold G. Wolff
Associate Professor of Medicine
Cornell Medical School
1300 York Avenue
New York, New York

Dear Dr. Wolff:

I plan to take residency training in Ophthalmology, and am particularly interested in Neuro-ophthalmology. I hope to receive this training under Dr. McLean at New York Hospital. I wrote Dr. McLean recently regarding the advisabilty of taking a year of Neurology prior to starting my residency in Ophthalmology, and he agrees that it would be excellent preparation.

Your service at Kingsbridge Veterans Hospital has been highly recommended to me by Dr. Foo Chu (Cornell '46). I would appreciate any information you could send me regarding the advisability and possibility of receiving a year of training there.

I expect to be released from the Navy during the first two weeks of July.

Thank you for your kind cooperation in this matter.

Very truly yours,

Edward W. D. Norton Lt.(jg) MC USNR
(Cornell '46)

LETTER TO HAROLD WOLFF FROM EWDN

we are not privy. But it is obvious from his letters to his mentors, Harold Wolff and John McLean, his plans were already formulated for his course of study in ophthalmology and neuro-ophthalmology. It is clear that he was planning to extend his professional training beyond residency in ways that were almost unheard of in that day.

Though with as yet no formal training in ophthalmology, he nevertheless received accolades from the men under whom he worked in the eye clinic at San Diego Naval Hospital.

And with that we close this chapter of his life. Discharged from active duty, it was time to begin formal preparation for his career. Circumstances seemed to rise to try his will, yet he met every one of them. And so the young family, Ed, Mary, Carol Ann and the new baby, Brian, born March 9, 1949, left San Diego in June of 1949 to return to New York Hospital and Cornell.

CHAPTER 6

Return to New York

1950 – 1953

By PRIOR ARRANGEMENT AND CONSENT FROM BOTH HAROLD WOLFF, Chairman of Neurology and John McLean, Chief of the Division of Ophthalmology, Ed began fifteen months as a resident in neurology. Although only twenty-eight, he was obviously able to impress his superiors that they were dealing with someone special.

Cornell, though not as stiff-backed as its Ivy League neighbor to the north, was nevertheless not what one would dub easygoing or flexible. The arrangement was for Ed to be based at the Kingsbridge VA hospital in the Bronx, then a satellite of Cornell. He had come highly recommended for the position by the Assistant Dean at Cornell.

The family was able to rent a ground floor flat in a triplex on King Avenue in Dunwoodie, a small village in Yonkers near the Knesniks. Ed was also able to see patients on the Cornell service in neurology at Bellevue Hospital, a veritable goldmine of neurological patient material.

During this interval he and Paul Wetzig (a name that will appear again and again in this work), produced a 16 mm film demonstrating the physical findings of oculomotor disorders of the visual system. The film ran almost an hour. Norton was the demonstrator of each patient's pathology and, when watching it, one could sense the man's exquisite attention to detail in examination (which remained a hallmark of his practice through the years). There were no shortcuts.

Wetzig was the cameraman, and the two edited the film together. They did the work on Saturdays and Sundays on their own time, as the clinical material was available. It remains a classic. And when Norton narrated the film, even years later, the memories of individual patients and their ocular problems were still vivid to him.

CORNELL UNIVERSITY MEDICAL COLLEGE
1300 YORK AVENUE
NEW YORK 21. N. Y.

January 15, 1949

Dr. Earl C. Gluckman, Director
Veterans Administration Hospital
150 West Kingsbridge Road
Bronx 65, New York

Dear Dr. Gluckman:

      Dr. Edward W. D. Norton, one of our graduates in the class of 1946, has asked me to submit a statement in support of his application for residency training in neurology at the Kingsbridge Veterans Hospital, beginning July 1, 1949.

      I am glad to commend Dr. Norton for serious consideration. In the undergraduate course at Harvard he made a very good record, placing on the dean's list in his third year. In the medical course he proved to be one of the top-rating students in his class. He placed in the first quarter of the class and was elected to the honorary medical society of Alpha Omega Alpha in his fourth year. In addition to this record of high scholarship, Dr. Norton has demonstrated excellent personal qualifications. He is quiet and agreeable in his work and a person who shows a very likeable nature.

                    Sincerely yours,

                    Dayton J. Edwards
                    Associate Dean

DJE:DBL
Transcript Enclosed.

LETTER TO KINGSBRIDGE VA HOSPITAL FROM CORNELL

Ed and Paul presented the film (as residents) at an AMA meeting in New York City in 1952 (the last time the AMA met in that city) and, though I have been unable to unearth documentation of this, I believe they won first prize for their efforts. The film was presented in many places over the years and is stored in the film archives of the Bascom Palmer Eye Institute.

The fifteen months on the neurology service flew by swiftly. Wolff was more than pleased with his unorthodox trainee and regretted that he had not been able to snare him for Neurology but rather had to release him to Ophthalmology.

We have very little evidence of Ed's record as one of Harold Wolff's residents at the Kingsbridge VAH. Beyond the accomplishment of producing the movie mentioned above, it is a rather silent gap in the record. We can speculate that the film was put together during 1950. In a sense it prefigured David Cogan's masterpiece, *The Neurology of Ocular Muscles*, published in 1956. (It is also interesting that Ed spent part of his post-residency fellowship year with Dr. Cogan, and the two became lifelong friends.)

Suffice it to say that there was never an instance within my recall when Ed Norton was stumped by a patient's motility disturbance, even if he didn't happen to recall the syndrome name. Starting from first principals, an intimate knowledge of the anatomy of the wiring of the brain, and a Sherlock Holmesian deductive ability, he could tell where to look for the lesion. He took a positive delight in it, as did his close colleagues of later years who loved to play "let's stump the Chief." It really illustrates, though, a subtler point about the man, namely the effort expended, the painstaking attention to detail he put forth.

What sort of man was he during this time? Busy, it goes without saying, but obsessed, no. An interesting vignette tells of a different sort of dedication. Janet Knesnik, Mary's "little sister" (whom we met in the last chapter) tells of missing school for three or four weeks due to an appendectomy. She was told by her geometry teacher (yes, they did teach subjects like that in American schools at the time) that she had better plan to repeat the year as there was no way she could pass the test. The busy doctor told her that there was no word for "can't" in his vocabulary and backed it up by tutoring her nightly. She received a grade of 92 on her Regents (New York's statewide examination).

Ed traveled to and from work by train and in cool weather wore earmuffs and overshoes and carried an umbrella. His sister-in-law interpreted that as a playfulness in him ("I think he liked to be a character"). Another interpretation that might fit with his aversion to the cold: his memories of childhood rheumatic fever and the long sojourns of bed rest that resulted from it.

Throughout the New York period, and although his schedule called for long hours of commitment, Mary contrived for him to make time available nights and weekends for her and the children. This often took the form of picnic suppers at Orchard Beach on City Island, not far from where they lived, or outings to the many parks that invest New York City.

> *To the surprise of many visitors, New York is not just bleak canyons of skyscrapers and grim granite buildings but also a city of many and varied parks; the best known, of course, is Central Park. These parks are thanks to the combined efforts of its politicians at the turn of the century, such as Theodore Roosevelt, who teamed up with Frederick Law Olmstead and Calvert Vaux, noted conservationists. (Would it, could it happen today?)*

With the combined efforts of the two parents, a family life for the Norton children, now numbering three with the birth of Mary Elizabeth (Marybeth) on January 3, 1951 (the same birthday as her dad), took shape and remains a vivid and very happy memory for Carol Ann.

⁓

Finished at the Bronx VA in October, 1950, Ed Norton again moved his family, this time to 1303 York Avenue, across the street from Cornell–New York Hospital, in preparation for beginning his residency in ophthalmology under John McLean.

CORNELL UNIVERSITY MEDICAL COLLEGE
1300 York Avenue
New York, N. Y.

January 15, 1950

Dr. Edward W. D. Norton
Veterans' Hospital
130 West Kingsbridge Road
Bronx, New York

Dear Dr. Norton:

Your recommendation for appointment to the resident staff in Ophthalmology at the New York Hospital has gone through. With this appointment there is also an appointment on the faculty of Cornell Medical College as Assistant in Ophthalmology.

Will you be good enough to fill out the enclosed blank and return it to me at your earliest convenience so that this appointment may also be put through. Your appointment will start October 1, 1950.

Very truly yours,

John M. McLean, M.D.

LETTER TO EWDN FROM JOHN MC LEAN

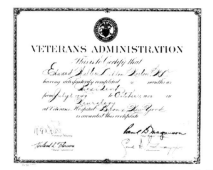

NEUROLOGY RESIDENCY CERTIFICATE, 10/1/50

But it was not to be, at least not yet. A routine examination diagnosed pulmonary tuberculosis and called for six months' hospitalization at NYH. There was something almost biblical in its message. Was not the good Lord trying the patience of His subject? All plans were on hold for at least six months while the man had to set down the tasks and goals to permit the healing of his body.

Carol Ann has a few recollections of her father's illness and of having to be skin-tested to be sure the rest of the family did not have the disease. She has a shadowy recall of visiting her father in the hospital in a "greenhouse" (?the solarium). He was in a bathrobe and sitting down, perhaps in a wheelchair (shades of the days of the stroller in childhood!).

Her single strongest recollection during this trying period is that a group of house staff led by Paul Wetzig got together and purchased a television set for the family, who were alone and perhaps under quarantine (remember these were the days of $25 to $50 per month stipends with laundry for house staff if you were lucky). A TV set was a luxury the family never could have purchased on their own.

Tuberculosis, formerly a death sentence to thousands in the teeming city slums, spawned by the Industrial Revolution, did not carry in 1951 quite the same ominous prognosis. The revolution in antibiosis, begun by Theodor Domagk at

*IG Farben in the Third Reich and continued by Sir
Alexander Fleming in Great Britain was in full swing in
the decade of the fifties. Streptomycin, isoniazid, and para-
amino salicylic acid were three chemotherapuetic agents
then available.*

*Certainly TB meant hospitalization, drug therapy with
annoying and occasionally serious side effects (hearing loss
with streptomycin), a rare resort to thoracic surgery in recal-
citrant cases, but on the whole the armamentarium of the
day had proven a match for the acid-fast bacillus that caused
caseating granulomas in tissues it colonized.*

But for a young physician, not quite thirty and with all the
gifts needed for a wonderful career in what seemed to be (and in
fact proved to be) the dawn of the golden age of medicine, it must
have been dismaying at least. Heartbreaking is perhaps a better word
when one remembers the rheumatic fever in childhood, and the
bulbar poliomyelitis of a few years later.

But with the same acceptance of the angel of illness that seemed
to sit on his shoulder, Ed Norton once again became the ward and
not the master of the health care system. He was hospitalized as an
inpatient on the tuberculosis ward at New York Hospital and all plans
to begin his residency training in ophthalmology were set aside.

He was released from the hospital six months later than his
planned start date; EWDN began as junior resident at the New York
Hospital–Cornell Medical Center in 1951. Living at the corner of
70th and York, he could literally walk across the street to work.

1303 York was an old fashioned, dark and somewhat gloomy
six story dwelling that seemed a veritable nest of John McLean's ophthalmology residents. It appeared that Miss Maloney, the silver-
haired icon of the Cornell housestaff housing office, saw to it
that there was always a good number of eye families to balance the

tense flock of general surgical residents in Frank Glenn's seven-year, pyramidal surgical program. Friendships with the more easygoing eye families were a welcome relief for some of them. On the other hand, all the physicians' families got on as only families in that peculiar state of equipoise can know. And somehow they do get through.

The ophthalmology program took one resident every nine months, so that three years later it had a senior resident with six months' experience.

When Ed began his residency, Paul Wetzig was his senior resident. Paul had interned at the Public Health Hospital in Staten Island and had been undecided

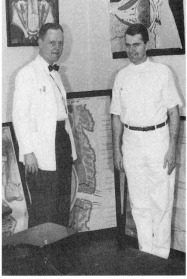

ED AND PAUL IN RETINA CLINIC

as to whether he should follow a career in otolaryngology or ophthalmology. Fortunately for all of us, John McLean offered him a position in the latter and the decision was made for him.

Paul and Dean Wetzig and their children, Carl and Dorreen (Dorrie), also lived at 1303 York. The Norton family now numbered three: Carol Ann, Brian and Marybeth. The Norton and the Wetzig children grew up together very much as their dads did professionally. Throughout the years to follow, the reunions of the families and their trips together—in Europe and this country—are the punctuation marks in the narrative cloth of their intertwined lives. Carol Ann remembers them fondly as the time the children had their fathers' attention fully and completely focused on nothing other than what was planned for today. And what a joy to have the undivided attention of those fathers!

At other times the dads were often on the brink of exhaustion from work and from sleep deprivation. And for the children, it was interminable waiting for the daddy who seems never to be able to come when he's counted on. Or planned outings cut short because the last patient seen on the ward before he left needed to have IVs changed in three hours; or six new admissions, wholly unscheduled, showed up and the on-call man was hollering for help.

> *Only those who have walked the walk and lived the life can grasp the delicate minuet, the balancing required to meet the conflicted needs for a physician and a family negotiating this hazardous passage a residency-training program had come to mean in this golden era of medicine.*
>
> *It took the tragic Libby Zion disaster at this same hospital some decades later to break the silence surrounding this "lifestyle" (if it can be called that) and force the whole story to the surface of public awareness.*
>
> *With all due respect to the Bell Commission report — recommending that residents work no more than 60 hours per week and that any resident working 24 hours had to have 24 hours off — it remains an open question whether any meaningful reform resulted from that episode, though a lot of ink was spent on it in the media.*

Outings together, planned or unplanned, babysitting duties traded, mutual support among and for the wives who were far more seriously isolated and alone than the men (medicine was for all practical purposes a consuming vocation and a strictly male preserve), and far more deprived than the more hyped "football widows" of later lore, their story of the costs of educating a husband and being in effect a single parent not on welfare, has yet to be told in any real way.

It is important to realize that John McLean's residency program was modeled closely on the Hopkins "sink or swim" model.

Residents, poorly prepared by anything they had learned in medical school or internship, were thrown into the clinic to learn pretty much on their own. Little time was spent in didactic learning from their elders, and attendings were a very scarce commodity in the clinic. And so the residents at New York Hospital developed a culture of resident education — by other residents.

> *I do not mean to disparage the system in so describing it, for it produced some wonderful ophthalmologists from a very, very, small program, Ed Norton being its prime exemplar. But it is obvious that Ed shaped his plans for his future pedagogy in reaction to the system. Even as a young attending he began to live outside that model.*

Ed Norton as a first year resident, because of his maturity and exposure to ophthalmology in the San Diego Naval Hospital outpatient eye clinic and to Meyer Wiener, MD, its civilian consultant, had a huge head start. A debt he always acknowledged.

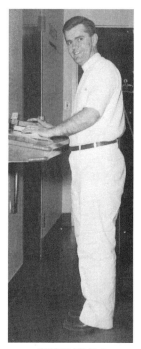

A picture of him from that era shows him going through the charts with a sly grin on his face. More than likely, knowing his voracious appetite for plain hard work, he had reserved the toughest and most interesting cases for himself.

What little we know of his residency years comes mostly from apocryphal tales told of "Doctor Norton," in hushed and reverential tones by Edna Carmen, RN, the eye nurse who ran the clinic on H-8 with her alter ego, Marian, the ageless clinic aide, to other, later, lazier residents who never could measure up to the man of the stories. It was, however, always difficult to disentangle whether the stories originated from his days as a resident or a young faculty member, the memories of the two women not dwelling on

EWDN IN H-8 CLINIC HALL

LEFT:
NOTE FROM A
PATIENT WHOM
EWDN OPERATED
ON AS A
RESIDENT

BELOW:
EWDN'S REPLY

March 3, 1992

Ms. ████████████
████████████████
████████████████

Dear Ms. ████████

I just received your delightful letter of February 26th. While you
may think that 39 years is too long a time for me to remember, I
can assure you that I remember the operation like it was yesterday.
At the time, I knew it was a difficult tumor to remove and to leave
you with an acceptable cosmetic result. After much consultation,
I did remove the tumor and repaired the drooping lid in a single
operation quite different than what had been the usual approach.
Postoperatively, I knew that we had been blessed by selecting the
right operation and having the Good Lord guide us.

Thank you for taking the time to send me your words of appreciation
I am enclosing under separate cover a copy of the history of Bascom
Palmer Eye Institute. I hope you have many years of health and
enjoyment. Thank you again.

Sincerely,

Edward W.D. Norton, M.D.
Chairman Emeritus
Leach Professor of Ophthalmology

EWDN/rcm

that distinction. Undoubtedly there was a grain or more of truth in them, but there had to be some exaggeration of the details in the retelling many times over.

We do have an indication, though, of the care he gave his patients as a resident. It is this sort of documentation of the care and the awareness of the care they received from him that lend credence to the stories of Edna and Marion, if any were needed.

Edward A. Dunlap, MD, John McLean's first recruit and the beloved teacher who trained all New York Hospital eye residents of the McLean era in ocular motility, was considerably more reserved about Ed's performance as a resident. "He was a good resident but nothing in his performance as a resident prefigured the brilliance of his later career."

Perhaps it was the contrast between how Norton, or any resident, can impress faculty as compared to Ed Norton's later deeds and accomplishments. Or perhaps it was that Ed Norton never played poker with Ed Dunlap after hours, as so many of his residents did.

Ed Norton and Ed Dunlap were, over the many years of their friendship, as close to one another as either of these very private men's personalities would permit. And when they got together, a certain amount of playful horseplay was called for ("you can take the boy out of high school . . .").

Ed Dunlap, Paul Wetzig and Vic Curtin were the closest of confidants as Edward Norton began his long quest for fulfillment of his dream. During his residency Ed had been already busy implementing his plan for post-residency education in ophthalmology.

During the fifties, post-residency training had not reached the level of acceptance and organization that it enjoys today. Planning for it depended on individual initiative to a great extent, which Norton had in great measure. Neuro-ophthalmology was his goal at this stage. There were really two places to go for a young man bent

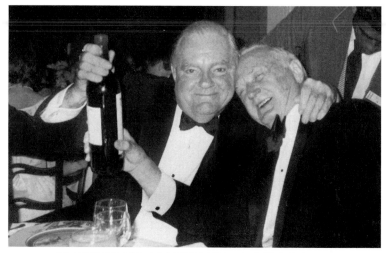

ED NORTON AND ED DUNLAP IN A LIGHTER MOMENT

on a career in that subspecialty: to Frank Walsh at Hopkins or Dave Cogan at Harvard. Why not both?

And so it was that Ed, finished with his residency at New York Hospital–Cornell Medical Center, prepared once again to leave his family for months, to pursue his now more-focused dream in Boston and Baltimore.

CHAPTER 7

Fellowship at Hopkins and Harvard: An Unplanned Encounter

1953

CHARLES DARWIN TELLS US FROM HIS RUMINATIONS ON EVOLUTION, "The survivors are not necessarily the strongest nor the brightest, but the most adaptable."

On its surface this seems almost a trivial observation given the significance of what his theory held for the human belief system that men held about themselves before it burst upon their consciousness. But on a subtler level it is full of meaning. Those living organisms that possessed the malleability to sense change by whatever means as it occurs, and adapt their behavior to its demands, are the ones who survive and propagate.

We now know that this adaptability inheres largely in our genes, unknown at the time to Darwin. Those organisms trapped in a rigid mold of any kind of behavior when change comes, perish. Ed Norton, though governed by an inflexible set of internalized principles in much of his behavior, was quintessentially the epitome of an adaptable organism in the deepest sense of which Darwin's aphorism applies.

The whole point of Norton's planned training up to now had turned on his fascination with the workings of the most complicated machine in the universe, the human mind, as it appeared through the workings of its physical realization, the brain. And it was the subtleties of the disordered workings of the mind-brain nexus, manifested in the visual system, that was his muse, as it was for both David Cogan and Frank Walsh, whom he had chosen as mentors.

These two men — the founding fathers of their specialty — were easily the best mentors he could have chosen in the US, if not the world. Both became fast friends with him. One had simply to witness in later years the respect and affection they had for him, their trainee — one of the first and undoubtedly among their very best. For their part, they genuinely loved Ed Norton.

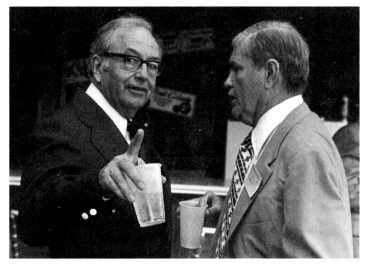

DAVID COGAN AND ED NORTON

Our understanding of the visual system, the most studied and familiar of the mind's (or brain's) subsystems, was beginning to take another wondrous leap, similar to the leap that characterized the work of Helmholtz and Hering and Sherrington in the nineteenth century. Names such as Kuffler and Hubel and Wiesel and Wald and Hecht and Polyak in the US, and Stiles and Crawford and Rushton and Weale in England, began to publish quantitative descriptions of its biology and even the physical equations that governed its performance.

Norton in no sense slighted his planned period of study with Cogan and Walsh. It was just that in Boston, at Massachusetts Eye and Ear Infirmary, he met a solitary, at times morose *Flamand,*

Charles Schepens. From Schepens he learned how to use the instrument he (Schepens) had brought with him from Belgium, the binocular indirect ophthalmoscope.

> *Schepens had come from Ghent, Belgium, the epicenter of Flemish culture and also the center of the peculiar (to our eyes and ears) mindset of these talented, secretive, almost devious appearing people who guard jealously what they consider theirs.*
>
> *Perhaps we can understand that a little better if we remember the eclipse of their civilization, Europe's dominant one at the time, occurred as that of their two powerful and unscrupulous neighbors, Germany and France, blossomed.*

Although not the inventor of the indirect ophthalmoscope, Schepens was for all practical purposes its popularizer and its leading proponent in this country. The line between the inventor and the advocate becomes blurred when one thinks of how long it might have lain dormant without Schepens' promotional skills.

Norton at once realized he had been given the tool that could make his brightest dreams come true. He learned, again primarily from Schepens but also from the small cadre of disciples attracted to him in spite of his singular and off-putting personality, how to examine the retina to find the break that Jules Gonin of Lausanne, Switzerland, had been describing as the cause of retinal detachments but which few could see with the existing instruments.

Finally, he learned the painstaking and later abandoned technique (by everybody in the field save Schepens) of scleral dissection, diathermy, and scleral implant with Polyviol tubing that Paul Custodis of Dusseldorf, West Germany had developed and taught Schepens before his journey to the US.

Norton recognized immediately the value of what he had been taught and changed course "on a dime," so to speak, to become a retina surgeon. Not at the expense of neuro-ophthalmology but rather in addition to it. The man's maturing intellect was such that two so very different disciplines could coexist easily in his mind.

Like every survivor in biological evolution, on some level he realized that change was coming in an area of ophthalmology that was, at the time, largely a hopeless dead-end: the surgery of retinal detachment. He would become an agent of the change that this new knowledge was bound to bring about in the largest city of the world.

His fifteen-month fellowship over, supported in part by a Heed stipend and monies from John McLean, Ed Norton returned to New York to begin his academic career and take the first tentative steps of his ascent where no man had gone before.

CHAPTER 8

Return to New York II
"The Only One in NYC Fixing Retinas"

1954 – 1957

ON HIS RETURN TO HIS FAMILY IN NEW YORK AND TO THE POSITION of instructor in Surgery (ophthalmology), Ed Norton was probably the best-trained and brightest ophthalmologist in the entire city. (He may or may not have been aware of it.)

It was the mid-fifties. John McLean was still very much the master surgeon in the city, but his department—with the exception of Ed Dunlap, Dan Gordon and Stuart Snyder—was thin. Columbia's Harkness Eye Institute boasted of stellar names such as Dunnington, Reese, Smelser, and later De Voe and many others. But that institution was already well along in the process of drawing its talent exclusively from within its own walls and never sending any of its "bright young men" for fellowships elsewhere.

> These young men became the junior partners of the older stars, and growth seemed to stop right there, a practice that was to have over the next decades a devastating effect on the evolution of that once dominant institution. The old standbys, the eye and ear infirmaries, Manhattan and New York, were training good clinical ophthalmologists but, lacking university affiliations, they could aspire to nothing beyond that task academically. The other academic affiliated programs were small and not on the level of Cornell and Columbia.

Ed Norton could do something that nobody else could at that time in New York City. He could (and did) fix a detached retina.

A record of the very first patient he treated, Mr. Charles Seitz, still exists, including his drawing of the retina and his note to the insurance company concerning the case. The two men met one another in follow-up some thirty-six years later with the retina still attached and the eye still seeing well at 20/30 acuity.

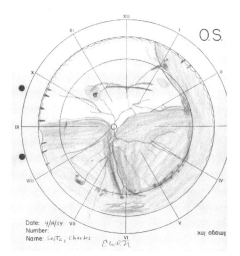

EWDN'S DRAWING OF CHARLES SEITZ'S RETINAL DETACHMENT

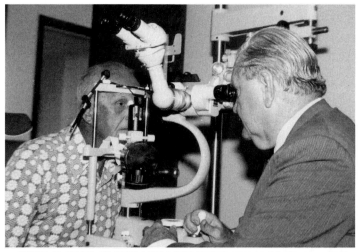

CHARLES SEITZ AT THE SLIT LAMP WITH EWDN 36 YEARS LATER

Within a very short period of time Edward Norton was "the man" to see in New York City if you had a retinal detachment. Word traveled quickly and patients soon filled the waiting area outside his tiny office.

What sort of man did they find? They met a man who radiated confidence without arrogance, intelligence without condescension, who had a genuine interest in their problem and an ability to communicate his commitment to find a solution if one existed.

Jaded New Yorkers were charmed by this humble yet very bright man. He won their confidence by his manner; he was every inch the

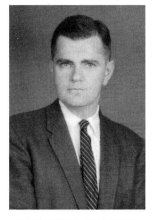

ED NORTON, NEW YORK HOSPITAL-CORNELL, 1956

physician he had trained himself to be. And it made no difference (as it never should in medicine) whether they came with the poorest of means or were from the elite celebrity strata, all were treated with the same care and respect, and all became his devoted patients because of it.

> *It happens not infrequently in medicine, if a physician has particular skills that somehow set him (or her) apart from their colleagues, their ego grows out of all proportion to the gift they possess. Perhaps it has to do with the ego every man or women needs to get through the arduous task of becoming a physician in the first place, or perhaps to the very unique effort called for to stand out from a very intelligent group of colleagues that form the medieval guild that is (or was) medicine. Whatever the reason, Ed Norton possessed none of it.*

One of Ed's most devoted patients, Harry Belafonte, had his retinal detachment repaired by Ed early in his career. Except for a transient double vision that disappeared without requiring further surgery, the repair was uneventful. Years later, as keynote speaker at an American Academy of Ophthalmology meeting, Belafonte acknowledged that his life had been changed by the encounter with Ed Norton. Besides being an entertainer, he has made the eradication of world blindness his life's work.

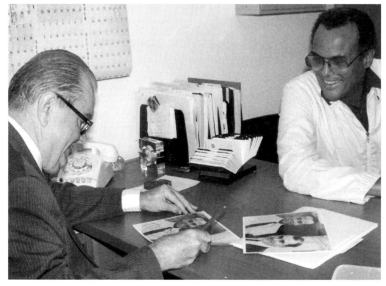

ED WITH HARRY BELAFONTE

An aspect in the Norton family life that changed on his return to New York and faculty status at NYH–Cornell was their financial circumstances. The Nortons moved to a garden apartment in Yonkers near the Knesniks. They now had a telephone (party line) but as yet no automobile.

During Ed's absences Mary, functionally a single parent with three small children, enrolled in evening courses at Columbia. Her being able to do so remains a source of amazement to Carol Ann after all these years, and a testimony to her mother's energy. Having grandparents nearby was undoubtedly very helpful.

After two years, the family was ready for still another move — to Rockne Road in Yonkers. It was the very first home the couple owned, a landmark in the married life of the day. Among its amenities it had three bedrooms! Always before, two bedrooms were all they could find in their price range.

> *The family now numbered four with the arrival of Kevin on March 8, 1958. It was during this period that the family took a trip to San Francisco at Dohrmann Pischel's invitation. On the way back they stopped off in Colorado Springs to see the Wetzigs; this began a series of reunions that were "a gift from both sets of parents to their children." The trips were cherished by all and were to continue until 1990.*

Rockne Road was apparently a delightful place to live. With a garden in the back, it was a welcome change for the children from the noisy, befouled atmosphere of York Avenue where a pitifully small, dingy concrete play yard at the back of 1303 was their "on site" recreation. Barring a trip to Central Park, which required one parent at least, it was the best the neighborhood could provide.

Carol Ann remembers a particularly telling incident that embodied her father's approach to leisure time with his children and the inquiring mind that guided all his activities.

Somehow he had decided that archery could become a family sport. Not satisfied with the usual "once over lightly" that such aberrations generally take in the paternal mind, followed quickly by recovery of common sense, Norton bought books, the requisite bows, and a quiver of arrows. A target was set up in the backyard, and for a period of undetermined length the family became Robin Hood and his Merry Band of Children-in-Training. For those of us who have witnessed the intensity with which he pursued winning a softball or tennis game, the vignette strikes a chord. These were, in all, happy and prosperous times for the family.

The Knesnik grandparents unwittingly opened another door. They had ventured south to Key West for a wintertime vacation (sometime before 1956) and reported back enthusiastically about their sojourn in the sun. They had stayed at a particular motel and become friendly with the owner and his wife. The Nortons followed in 1956. Taking the children out of school, they all piled in the family car and made the trip an adventure.

In the dreary, long, cold winter, to get out of school (even with schoolbooks and study schedule brought along) and go to that lovely, balmy winter-in-South Florida climate was a delight! And well deserved after the long separations that they had endured without murmur or complaint.

Still another thread in the life of the man at that time deserves comment: the impact of his return to NYH on the academic life of the program there. Indeed, the level of teaching picked up at many New York institutions just because Norton raised the bar at Cornell.

As Tom Kearns, one of his junior residents recalls, "Norton was arrow straight, a great teacher, athletic, competitive, and honest to the core. His innate strength to help and support others is known to all. I honestly believe he taught Arnold Palmer the meaning of the word charisma." A true southern gentleman's appraisal of his faculty mentor of 40 years before.

Established practitioners, potential competitors such as Harvey Lincoff, came to hear his lectures. "I learned what I know of neuro-ophthalmology from Ed Norton" was a statement he made to the author some years later, and Lincoff is not effusive in his praise of anybody.

Norton continued to be not just the teacher, but also the student. Years later he acknowledged his debt to the lectures of Alfred Kestenbaum, the old world–trained refugee neuro-ophthalmologist. Kestenbaum gave a yearly series of lectures at night at New York

Eye and Ear Infirmary. These later appeared in print in his book *Clinical Methods of Neuro-Ophthalmological Examination*, published in 1946, now out-of-print, but a gem.

> *A practical and pragmatic physician, part of the duo that independently, but in the same year, in widely separated parts of the globe, originated the operation for nystagmus that bears their names as the Kestenbaum-Anderson (or Anderson-Kestenbaum in the Southern Hemisphere). Professor Kestenbaum had a penchant, nay a facility, for setting up rules and algorithms (for his time far advanced) for neuro-ophthalmological diagnosis. Ed Norton appreciated that organizing skill wherever he found it.*

The situation for Norton at New York Hospital–Cornell could not remain in equilibrium for long, however. The young faculty member was just too good a physician and his practice grew apace as a result. In the few short years he was there, his was the busiest practice in the division.

For reasons that remain a mystery to all who knew him, John McLean never pushed the issue of departmental status for Ophthalmology, to which he and the entire faculty were well entitled, particularly with the addition of Norton. Pioneering work in uveitis had been done with ACTH and cortisone shortly after its debut by McLean and Gordon. McLean was universally respected by his colleagues in the specialty, as was Ed Dunlap in ocular motility. Ophthalmology had produced for its small size an unusual number of outstanding young clinicians who were making a name for themselves. Yet McLean demurred.

The situation came to a head in what Dunlap describes with relish as "Cornell's 120-square-foot-mistake." At a loss to know how, or rather where, to put the horde of waiting patients whenever he saw them, Norton had requested from administration a 10- by 12-foot space to be taken from the Benson Optical Shop's premises.

Because of the divisional status of the eye service the request had to go through Frank Glenn, the Louis Atterbury Stimson Professor and Chairman of the Department of Surgery, and the real power at New York Hospital and Cornell in clinical matters even as trivial as this.

> *With the change in chair, Medicine dropped from its former exalted status at NYH to a rather lackluster one. Surgery definitely had the upper hand in this eternal and largely unnecessary turf battle between these two backbone services.*

Frank Glenn turned Norton's request down cold, advancing the rather lame excuse that if he gave space to the eye service, ENT would not be far behind, and besides the optical shop was producing revenue for "the department" and that revenue was somehow critical to the program.

The die was cast. After an unsuccessful attempt to find suitable quarters in one of the office buildings near the hospital, Ed resolved that his destiny lay elsewhere, the elsewhere to be filled in later.

And so, on the cold, gray, blustery morning of November 27, 1957, riding up in the G building elevators of NYH, John McLean casually (he always seemed most casual at such times) mentioned to Ed Norton that he had recently received a letter from some program in South Florida looking for a man to run it.

We can only imagine the thrill that went through his young colleague's mind. As diffident and shy a man as McLean was, he probably completely misread Norton's interest in seeing the letter. If ever there was an appropriate place for that overused aphorism "the right man at the right time." And the rest is history.

CHAPTER 9

South Florida and the Founding of Bascom Palmer

1958 – 1965

IN THE MYSTERIOUS WAYS FATE HAS OF PREPARING US FOR OUR destiny, all of Ed Norton's life seemed to have been pointing to South Florida in general and Miami in particular. His early childhood vacations where for the first time he felt healthy, learned to swim and could enjoy the warm water and the sun, to the trips when he and Mary and the children returned for winter sojourns.

How did it come to be that John McKenna wrote to John McLean, Chief of the Division of Ophthalmology (and many other program professors) at the right time — soon after Surgery's denial of Norton's request at NYH — and to the right man? We will never know. But we do know that Ed Norton answered with alacrity if not betraying a hint of eagerness.

There followed over the ensuing months the delicate dance over the particulars of the position that takes place between the candidate and the search committee, which seems to have consisted of one man, John J Farrell, MD, Chairman of Surgery — all of which has to be agreed to by the Dean, Homer Marsh, PhD.

Ophthalmology was a division of Surgery (shades of NYH). There is one letter of surpassing interest—Ed Norton's letter to Dr. Farrell on his (Ed's) conditions that had to be met for him to take the job; its first page is printed here. (The complete text is available in the archives of Bascom Palmer.) This missive must rank among

UNIVERSITY OF MIAMI
SCHOOL OF MEDICINE
JACKSON MEMORIAL HOSPITAL
MIAMI 36, FLORIDA

DIVISION OF OPHTHALMOLOGY

November 21, 1957

J. McLean, M. D.
New York Hospital
New York City, New York

Dear Dr. McLean:

I am in the rather sad position of looking for a successor and am taking the liberty of writing to you to see if you know of anyone you might suggest. Our new medical school, which has now graduated two classes, has definitely decided on a program of constructing each division with a chief who must be a salaried individual, geographically full-time in the hospital, with a right to a limited amount of consultation practice only. I, on the other hand, being in the private practice of ophthalmology in this community, have been organizing the Division on a part-time basis, and my situation is therefore temporary.

An applicant for the position as Chief of the Division of Ophthalmology should be someone who has indicated clearly he has decided to remain permanently in academic medicine, who would be interested in and qualified to handle the combination of administrative and teaching duties, and, of course, inaugurating and supervising the usual investigative programs. He should probably be an individual of some maturity and experience beyond the usual three year resident level although the latter qualification is not absolute.

We have already undergone a good deal of organizational activity. Our residency is approved for a full three years, and we now have four residents and appropriations to include a total of six from next year on. Because the site of the school, Jackson Memorial Hospital, is a large general hospital, we have a wealth of clinical material, and because there is a private component to the hospital and a growing clinical faculty of interested and capable attending ophthalmologists, we have additional surgery for the residents to assist with and good attendance and cooperation by the visiting men. The hospital is now about to build three hundred additional beds of which one floor of about thirty beds will be devoted to white adult eye patients, and we have, in addition, access to as many colored and pediatric beds as we need.

PAGE 1 OF A LETTER TO JOHN MC LEAN FROM JOHN MC KENNA,
IN SEARCH OF A CHIEF FOR THE DIVISION OF OPHTHALMOLOGY

November 29, 1957

Dr. John F. McKenna, Chief
Division of Ophthalmology
University of Miami School of Medicine
Jackson Memorial Hospital
Miami 36, Florida

Dear John:

In line with our telephone conversation of
November 28, I am forwarding to you a summary of my background, training, present appointments, society member-
ships, publications and lectures. I shall close with a
brief list of what I would like to consider as my accomplishments.

If the University of Miami School of Medicine is
interested in considering me for the position as Chief of
the Division of Ophthalmology, I would like to discuss
the situation further with the proper authorities.

Incidentally, I do not have a Florida license,
so if I am considered seriously for the position I would
appreciate hearing soon so that I can take the necessary
steps to acquire one.

Sincerely yours,

Edward W. D. Norton, M. D.

EWDN:sjs

LETTER TO JOHN MC KENNA FROM EWDN, APPLYING FOR THE POSITION

January 23, 1958

Dr. John J. Farrell
Chairman, Department of Surgery
University of Miami School of Medicine
Jackson Memorial Hospital
Miami 36, Florida

Dear Dr. Farrell:

I was pleased to receive your letter of January 13th offering me the
position of Chief of the Division of Ophthalmology of the University
of Miami School of Medicine and the Chief of Ophthalmology at the
Jackson Memorial Hospital.

From the extensive talks I had with you, Dean Marsh and Dr. Gates
during my recent visit to Miami I have evolved a group of conditions
which I would like to set forth as a basis for my accepting your
offer. It is my understanding that we discussed all these conditions
and that they were mutually agreed upon verbally.

1) I will be promoted to full Professor of Ophthalmology,
at a salary of $12,000 a year, with the University
contributing an additional ten percent ($1,200)
annually into a retirement fund for me, at the end of
one year if I have shown promise in developing the
division of ophthalmology. In addition to the $12,000
salary I will be allowed to make an equal amount
from referred private practice.

2) I will receive tenure one year after my appointment
as full Professor.

3) It is the intention of the University of Miami School
of Medicine to make some sort of arrangement so that
the following tax-deductible expenses will be paid out
of earnings over and above the allowed amount:
   a) malpractice insurance premiums
   b) expenses to medical meetings
   c) purchase of medical books and journals
   d) entertainment of visiting members of the medical
      profession
   e) incidental expenses incurred from private practice

LETTER TO J.J. FARRELL FROM EWDN, ACCEPTING
POSITION AND LISTING CONDITIONS (PAGE 1)

UNIVERSITY OF MIAMI

SCHOOL OF MEDICINE

JACKSON MEMORIAL HOSPITAL

MIAMI 36, FLORIDA

DEPARTMENT OF SURGERY

February 5, 1958

Edward W. D. Norton, M.D.
525 East 68th Street
New York, New York

Dear Doctor Norton

I have gone over your letter of January 23, 1958 in considerable detail and
it would appear to me that the appropriate way to answer it is merely to refer to
the item numbers which you have specified in that letter. It is perfectly apparent
that it is impossible to spell out any contractual relationship that would go into
the very considerable detail taken up in your letter of January 23. It is also
obvious that mutual trust and confidence has to be expressed between individuals
and institutions as well as between individuals and other individuals involved
in the same medical school development. Now to refer to specific paragraphs.

1) As I stated in conversation it would be my intention to recommend such
advancement through proper administrative channels if the stipulations as specified
relative to the development of the division were fulfilled. Obviously no departmental
chairman carries the right in a University to actually carry out such promotions.
The departmental chairman can only recommend to his Executive Faculty and to his
Dean for further recommendations to the President of the University. The question
of salary and retirement fund as well as the amount received in a referred private
practice are part of the contract of the University before a man is accepted.

2) It is a policy of this University as stipulated in their contracts that
full professors obtain tenure in one year's time, associate professors two years
and assistant professors three years.

3) The plan of fringe benefits is still in the development stage down here
and it is impossible to specify all the possible ramifications of it when no such
plan has been officially adopted. The things that you have mentioned have been
discussed and there would appear to be considerable agreement on them.

d) Entertainment of visiting members of the medical profession is going
to have to receive considerable scrutiny on a medical school wise basis in order
to prevent the development of abuses. Just what mechanisms will be set up rests
with ultimate decisions of the Executive Faculty. My committee charged by the
Executive Faculty with drawing up the income plan for referred private practice
have in general considered and made recommendations on the things that you mentioned.
However, we are setting it up on a departmental basis as far as the acquisition of
some of the things you have mentioned and not on an individual basis of utilization
of the persons own funds for himself as such. In other words our basic agreement
between the Board of Trustees of the University, the Medical School itself and the

LETTER TO EWDN FROM J.J. FARRELL,
ACCEPTING CONDITIONS (PAGE 1)

the most astonishing a surgeon-chairman has ever received from any candidate for the Chair in Ophthalmology, traditionally one of the smallest and quietest of the subspecialties.

Norton's letter, when read carefully, clearly shows the effect of the lessons learned at NYH from his four-year sojourn there. Lessons of omission and commission. None of his conditions are unreasonable and three were non-negotiable. Without them Norton would have never achieved what he did over the next decades:

- Departmental status within one year;

- The building of an eye institute with departmental funds;

- Retention of departmental earnings within the department.

The letter is a masterpiece and could well be pondered by any young soul considering the decision to assume the thankless task that a department chair has come to mean today. Needless to say, the letter displayed all of Norton's ability to organize and prioritize the items on this agenda and then some. Dr. Farrell had undoubtedly never encountered the likes of Norton before — few people had.

By now Norton was in real possession of the means to his dream. He was all the more formidable in negotiations because of it. Fortunately, Dr. Farrell did not climb up on his high horse and do the usual surgical number on him but instead had the good sense to accede to most of Ed's conditions, at least in principle.

That was all Norton needed. He promptly accepted the position and began the arrangements to move his family to Miami and recruit his first faculty member, which proved a pivotal choice for him and the institution he was to found.

In his reply, Dr. Farrell counseled patience on the part of his applicant. Little did he realize the plans that Norton had in mind once he had achieved departmental status.

⁓

But we must break with his story here to describe the medical community as it existed in Miami in 1958. A fledgling medical school had graduated its first class in 1956. Needless to say, this had been a risky undertaking. Miami was largely a tourist town with no heavy (or light) industry as its backbone. Though it had wealthy people among its residents, these were largely part-time residents who fled the city in the long, hot and humid summer.

The medical school, at the time, was a cash sink, not a cow. Medicare would not be enacted for another seven years. Did the school possess sufficient staying power to survive? Although we know the answer today, that must have been one of the imponderables in 1958. The ophthalmological community, if it can be called that, consisted of a small group of practitioners, all in private practice, all from elsewhere.

Bascom Palmer, MD, had been the most prominent of them. He was, by virtue of his position in the community, also a member of the board of directors of the Miami Lighthouse for the Blind. The board had appropriated $200,000 to establish an eye clinic. In Dr. Palmer's words, its goals were to provide

- eye care for indigents and others.
- treatment and research.
- conservation of sight.
- dissemination of information.

Little did he or any of the members of that body realize how well his goals would be fulfilled by the man just chosen to head the Bascom Palmer Eye Institute. And all for $200,000! Bascom Palmer died in 1955; it was at his widow's urging that the new institute be named for her beloved husband.

Prior to Ed Norton's coming, the ophthalmological division of the Department of Surgery was headed by John McKenna (a private practitioner in Coral Gables) as acting chief of service. It had an approved residency with five residents in the program, a voluntary faculty consisting of essentially all the private practitioners in the community, an outpatient clinic, and a scattering of hospital beds throughout the racially segregated Jackson Hospital. This was the scene when Edward W.D. Norton, MD, the new full-time chief of service in Miami arrived in July of 1958.

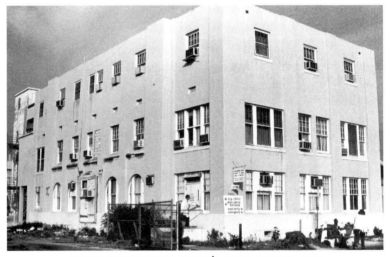

BUILDING HOUSING EWDN'S FIRST OFFICE, 1958

What about those left behind in New York City? An apocryphal story concerns John McLean. To say that he was disappointed to lose his brightest pupil would be an understatement. A good deal of his academic program left along with Ed Norton. McLean is said to have remarked that he (Norton) would be wasting his time in Miami. (Even the brilliant among us can have trouble seeing an opportunity when it stares us in the face.)

And the passing of Norton from the New York ophthalmological scene left a "hole" never filled by another like him.

The family made the journey to Miami that summer of 1958.

Ed had gone before in March and had rented a house that proved to be the only misstep in the whole logistical operation. When he and Mary called on the landlady for the key, with the family in tow, they discovered she had changed her mind.

Homeless in Miami: what to do? They found another real estate agent and rented another house — two houses in fact—on Crystal Court, where they lived until their permanent home was built.

> *When one thinks of the care the Nortons, particularly Mary, expended later in seeing that their faculty was well and quickly settled, I am sure that the solicitude echoed their past experience in the fragile rental market of Miami.*

At almost the same time, Ed purchased from Rance Riddle, MD, a former New York Hospital resident of an earlier vintage, a prime piece of property on the corner of South Bayshore Avenue and Emathla Street in Coconut Grove, to be the site of their future home. He engaged the services of a struggling young architect, Peter Jefferson, who was a kindred spirit to the young couple. "The easiest people I ever had to deal with — and the couple that gave me a start in the business."

> *Today, Peter is one of the nation's foremost designers for the people who build homes where price is no object. He speaks even now of the Nortons as intimate friends who participated in every phase of the design of their unique house.*

The house had jalousie windows and no air conditioning. Each room seemingly opened to and blended with the tropical surround and each had a view of the bay. During every stage of its construction, Ed would visit the site in the evening after work and delight in following the progress of the work (much as he was to do in later years with the other construction projects he undertook). Somewhere in his makeup was a builder (grandfather, a bricklayer)—how else to explain his keen interest and uncanny ability to read blueprints and pick out the tiniest design flaws missed by trained architects and draftsmen?

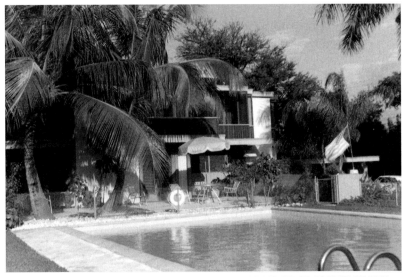

THE NORTON HOME AT 2121 S. BAYSHORE DRIVE IN COCONUT GROVE

Jefferson and the Nortons partied together, even (he recalls with relish) with the armaments minister of the government of Anastasio Somoza, the puppet El Presidente of Nicaragua. The minister (undoubtedly on a mission to protect the security and democracy of Nicaragua) brought his mistress along. The woman was absolutely charmed by Norton, who was completely oblivious of her obvious overtures. The other partygoers were not; one woman with a reasonable facsimile of an Hispanic accent was prevailed upon to call Ed in his office and ask for "a special appointment with him personally to check a blemish in her eye." At this point Ed's survival instincts kicked in and he quickly arranged to have her seen by someone else on the staff. All this was much to the merriment of the group.

Patti Norton Laird (born May 19, 1960), Ed and Mary's youngest daughter, informs me that the house — which holds fond memories for so many of the people, great and small, who, in passing through Bascom Palmer, enjoyed its warmth and open hospitality — is today in the hands of other owners. Though they have made changes to its exterior they have left its interior relatively unchanged, with that wonderful sense of space and openness Jefferson and the Nortons were able to capture in its design.

In the course of that first year (1958–59), a sixth resident was added, dedicated operating room time was established in the Jackson ORs, and weekly grand rounds were inaugurated—an academic highlight for the entire community—and Saturday morning teaching conferences were instituted. These conferences, as Victor Curtin (Ed's first faculty recruit, noted for his droll New England humor) put it in his Norton Lecture of 1996, "were instituted probably to the distress of the residents as it took thirty-three years and a new chairman to get them rescheduled during the week."

Over the resistance of the Chair of Surgery (they never change, do they?) departmental status was achieved in 1959 with the support of the dean, who was keenly aware that denial meant immediate resignation of the Chief of Ophthalmology. Ed Norton could play hardball when he needed to, but it was decidedly not his style.

Victor Curtin, in so many ways Ed Norton's alter ego, joined the faculty in 1959. Vic had been trained under Ed at NYH and followed him in his interest in retinal surgery. At Ed's behest he trained, post-residency, in retina at the Mass. Eye and Ear, and in pathology at the Armed Forces Institute of Pathology, and brought that subspecialty, so necessary in the training of young ophthalmologists, with him to Miami.

Between them, these two men displayed—in their differences in temperament, similarities in character and integrity—the full range of the Irish character. Each knew what the other was thinking on any given issue without the need to exchange words.

In the goal they set themselves, and in their selfless dedication to the task of making the BPEI the very best they could, the two men witnessed the truth of Loyola's words concerning character. They sought nothing for themselves. And all who came in contact with them were inspired by their example to do the same: to be the very best they could and to be part of something beyond themselves, to make a whole that would be greater than the sum of its parts.

Events moved swiftly. The Bascom Palmer Eye Institute building, begun in 1959, extended into 1960. Jackson Memorial Hos-

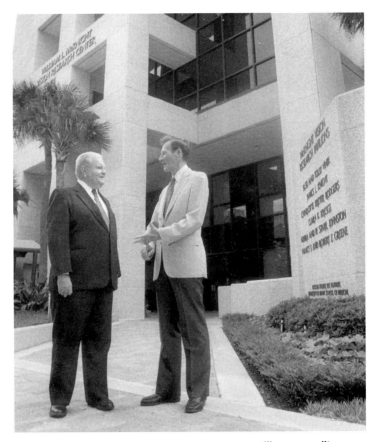

EWDN AND VTC OUTSIDE MC KNIGHT ("OLD BPEI")

pital expanded over the same time frame with the completion of the south wing, and Ophthalmology consolidated its in-patient beds at forty on South Wing 4. Space became available for the faculty offices, and air conditioning followed. Two examining rooms were added as well. Operating rooms, also two in number, became available on 4 Central.

When plans for Bascom Palmer were ready and submitted for bids, the low bid was $510,000. Since only $300,000 was in hand, a benefactor was needed. Kenneth Whitmer, MD, one the earliest and most steadfast friends of the institution throughout his life, interceded. Whitmer approached Mr. Claude Hemphill about the problem and opened the door for Ed Norton. Hemphill became the angel, the first of many. His donation permitted construction to proceed on schedule early in 1961. The building was completed in ten months and dedicated in January of 1962.

A few words are in order here about the building, and the foresight in its design implied. Four floors were built, the top one as a shell floor. The foundation would support eight (its present incarnation). This was typical of the Norton style: build for today but design for future needs as well. The structure contained private and resident examining rooms on its first two floors, and waiting rooms on the first floor.

The waiting rooms were embellished by a striking mosaic titled "The Woman at the Window." Thorne Shipley, PhD, the second of Ed Norton's recruits, headed the selection committee. The work was created by Miguel Duran-Lorega and Jesus Martitegui of Madrid, who won the design contest from among many entries. It was another hallmark of the care and love that went into the planning of the structures that, over the years, came to house the department—always to have some mark to celebrate the role that vision plays in relaying images of the beautiful and the true to our consciousness, amidst the otherwise mundane surround of an eye

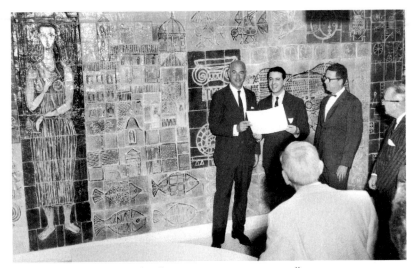

DEDICATION OF "WOMAN AT THE WINDOW" MOSAIC.
CLAYTON CHARLES, CHAIR OF THE ART DEPT. (L) AND
THE SPANISH COUNSUL IN MIAMI (R) ARE PICTURED.

clinic. It remains a memorable sight to all who enter the "old BPEI" for whatever reason, and most strongly to those residents, fellows and faculty of the pre-1976 era.

By 1962, outpatients were seen at the old Bascom Palmer Eye Institute. Beds available at Jackson Memorial Hospital. The eye department flourished. With growth in the physical plant, growth in the faculty continued apace. Each man was recruited differently, in a way tailored to his personality and a shrewd assessment of it by the new chairman. By 1965 the first edition of the "Wall Docs" was complete.

Each of the stories of the recruiting of those who created the backbone of the clinical faculty is a tale in itself. J. Lawton Smith, MD—the one and only JLS—arrived in 1962. His account of being recruited by Ed Norton from Duke contains elements of

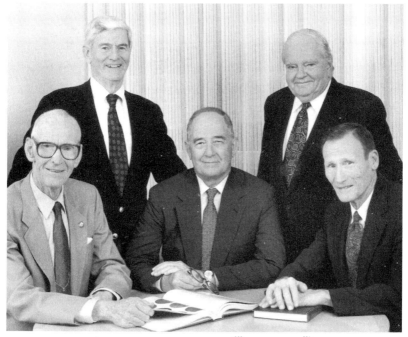

THE FOUNDING FATHERS ("WALL DOCS")

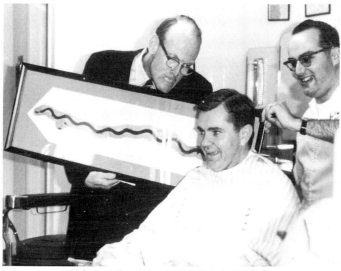

EWDN AND JLS IN A PLAYFUL MOMENT

high comedy as well as drama (available in archives) as one would expect of that unique individual.

Norton's impact on the academic life of the medical campus, indeed on the entire university, had been singular. He had detected signs of mental instability in a departmental chair and advised the man's quiet removal. Unfortunately his advice was ignored (not the last such occurrence during Norton's career in Miami) and the University had to endure the negative publicity when that unfortu-

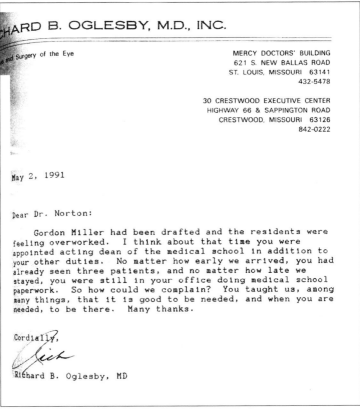

CHARD B. OGLESBY, M.D., INC.

and Surgery of the Eye

MERCY DOCTORS' BUILDING
621 S. NEW BALLAS ROAD
ST. LOUIS, MISSOURI 63141
432-5478

30 CRESTWOOD EXECUTIVE CENTER
HIGHWAY 66 & SAPPINGTON ROAD
CRESTWOOD, MISSOURI 63126
842-0222

May 2, 1991

Dear Dr. Norton:

      Gordon Miller had been drafted and the residents were feeling overworked. I think about that time you were appointed acting dean of the medical school in addition to your other duties. No matter how early we arrived, you had already seen three patients, and no matter how late we stayed, you were still in your office doing medical school paperwork. So how could we complain? You taught us, among many things, that it is good to be needed, and when you are needed, to be there. Many thanks.

Cordially,

Richard B. Oglesby, MD

LETTER TO EWDN FROM AN EARLY BPEI RESIDENT

nate's behavior resulted in commission of a crime.

On retirement of the Dean (in 1991), Homer Marsh, the man chosen to be acting Dean was of course Edward Norton. His tenure in the position, which was offered to him full time had he wanted it, was short: six months. During that short span he accomplished two major changes in the structure of the school that paved the way for its growth. These were:

a) independence of the medical school from the quasi control of the Dade County Medical Association, accomplished through amicable negotiation.

b) separation of academic rank from salary and from salary support. Without this, salary for each rank was fixed and supplemental income was limited to an amount equal to that fixed salary. With this separation, reward for academic achievement could occur and basic and clinical departments could achieve their own level of excellence, which they proceeded to do.

Norton, who had no desire for the office in the first place, chaired the search committee to find a suitable Dean and soon came back to his life's work, his growing department.

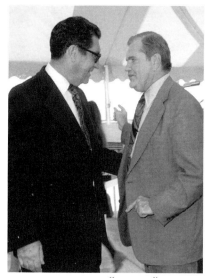

His dealings with the other deans during his chairmanship were always characterized by mutual respect, open mindedness, and open handedness. Emanuel (Manny) Papper, MD, Dean from 1969 to 1981 recalls, "I valued his counsel very much. His advice was always the kind that I cherished. It was optional and never directive; he would usually give me two or three or more suggestions or options and it was my responsibility to choose among them.

ED NORTON AND "MANNY" PAPPER

"Another episode that was important to me: When Mary Norton died, it was very tragic and a sad time for Ed and those close to him. He bore the loss with great fortitude, which is not necessarily a virtue, but in him, who was given to warmth of feeling and not being embarrassed by demonstration of emotion, it was singular to watch him continue with his major work in life."

Manny, like almost all who worked with Ed during those years of growth, worried a great deal about how much he cared for his own health. "That never seemed a high priority to Ed Norton."

Bernie Fogle, MD, his last Dean, echoed Papper's sentiments and added: "In 1976, before I became Dean, it came up in discussions that there were people who wanted to secede from the University, not pay taxes; the university connection was an albatross. It was Ed Norton who spoke up finally and quietly said, 'free-standing medical schools don't mean a whole heck of a lot—it would be an apprentice school; it really doesn't make sense,' and people did listen."

"Between indirect costs and taxation on the PIP, the department was giving the school in rent and other subsidies 2.7 million dollars a year and they only got back only 900,000 dollars. It was 3 to 1—a good deal for the school."

The new president of the University of Miami, Henry King Stanford, had occasion to interview Norton early in his tenure. He asked the question college presidents typically ask their department chairs: "What are your goals for your department?"

One can almost hear this avuncular, courtly southern gentleman from Americus, Georgia, asking it, perhaps adding "young man," perhaps not. He was wholly unprepared for the answer. "To build here at the University of Miami the best eye department in the country." At that moment he enlisted the man who would become his number one backer within the university bureaucracy for all the years they worked together, to achieve that aim.

Marshall M. Parks, MD, on a flight back east from a meeting in Kansas City he and Norton had attended, questioned the relatively unknown Norton about his goals in Miami. Norton took the occasion to outline in specific detail just what his plan was. The only question he could think to ask was "Ed, how in the world are you going to pay for it all?" Without a hint of hesitation Norton replied, "We are going to earn the money ourselves to pay for it." Decades later, Parks could only shake his head with friendship and admiration and say, "And by God he did."

With his faculty nucleus, and his teaching program designed to remedy all the defects he knew so well at NYH in place, the institution began to prosper academically. It also did well financially because he plowed excess earnings back into the department to build its financial base.

An eye bank, under the direction of Vic Curtin and supported by the Florida Lions, was established. It was and, as far as I am aware, still remains unique in charging no fee for providing the donor material and the service to recipients. This practice makes all other eye banks not just nervous but at times hostile. Knowing the single-minded dedication and unashamed altruism of these two men, it could not be otherwise.

Neuro-ophthalmology was already gaining national attention with names such as Noble David added to the neurology and the ophthalmology faculty. "Nobby" as he was known, came from Duke. He brought with him a little known method of angiography, using fluorescien dye to visualize the retinal vessels. (He also brought Johnny Justice, a young ophthalmic photographer who added a zest, if any was needed, to all conferences in which ophthalmic photography played a role—which was in fact practically all such conferences).

The department sponsored the first annual neuro-ophthalmology conference solely on this topic to be held in the United States.

Organized by Lawton Smith, its faculty listed David Cogan, Frank Walsh, Bill Hoyt and Hans Newton, among others. It proved to be an irresistible attraction to ophthalmologists and neurologists from the frozen northern climes in February. And it remained so for many years.

On another more subtle, but in many ways more important, level the program's praises were being touted by the residents as the best kept secret around; Miami was becoming the "in" place to be. Soon BPEI was competing with Wilmer, Mass. Eye and Ear, Wills and Columbia's Harkness Eye Institute for the best and brightest, and coming away with their share.

Ed Norton had envisioned from the first a department in which basic research prospered alongside the clinic and the two cross-fertilized each other. To this end he began recruiting basic science faculty to add to his growing nucleus of clinicians. The first was Thorne Shipley, PhD, a scholar of universal and diverse

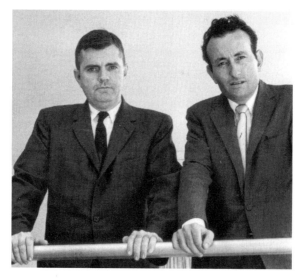

THORNE SHIPLEY AND ED NORTON

interests, among which were color and binocular vision. Thorne founded and for many years edited the journal *Vision Research*, with help from Reva Hurtes, BPEI's librarian. It is arguably the pre-eminent publication in this field today.

Thorne recalled somewhat wistfully the early days of grand rounds, when vision scientists and clinicians freely interacted and exchanged insights, and afterward all enjoyed a sandwich lunch in Ed's office.

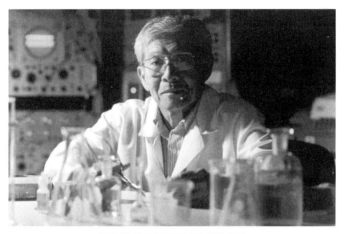

DUCO HAMASAKI IN HIS LAB

Ed's second recruit in the basic sciences was Duco Hamasaki, PhD. Duco, after finishing his optometry studies and doctorate under Gerald Westheimer at UC Berkeley, joined Giles Brindley for a post-doctoral year at Cambridge University in England. Ed, who was on the National Institute of Health's study section in vision, received Duco's application and recruited him by letter without ever meeting him. This was I believe unique in Norton's method of gathering his faculty. But then Duco is unique as well.

Since Duco joined the faculty in 1963, over two hundred post-doctoral students have passed through his laboratory. He has re-coded ERGs from almost one hundred twenty species of vertebrate and invertebrate retinas. Countless residents and medical students, undergraduate and even bright high school students (including my son) have learned about how science is done from this gentle man.

Describing his first encounter with Ed Norton: "He seemed like a very nice man, regular . . . he asked me what I needed . . . I said an office and some lab space and he provided me with them on the third floor . . . and within a month I was doing experiments. I noticed the man was here continuously, late at nights. I would walk out and see that VW bus parked, and early in the morning the bus was still there. He always said to me that he and the department were behind my research and if funds became scarce the department would support me."

There began in the sixties a series of trips to Europe with Paul Wetzig, to explore the latest developments in clinical retinal work coming from the Old World. Europe was ahead of the US in the field, particularly with the development of the xenon-arc photo-coagulator by Gerd Meyer-Schwikerath in Essen, West Germany. Ed secured the second instrument delivered in this country through the generosity of Paul, who lent his to BPEI and waited for BPEIs instrument to come later.

> *The sixties trip with Paul, recalled Carol Ann, caused tears on Mary's part at the airport on being left alone with five children for a month, probably six weeks. These were the days without cell phones, transatlantic calls were difficult to place and expensive and mail from Europe problematic at best. It couldn't have been easy.*

A major hurricane, Donna, hit Miami during the early fall. Kevin was age three. Many years later he recalled the storm and its aftermath in a lyrical essay he titled Bayshore Dreams. "Giant coconut trees, and ficus and gumbo-limbo were thrashing and bent almost parallel to the ground, while all manner of seaside debris flew horizontally across his field of vision at terrific speeds. The wonderful new house snuggled atop the bluffs on Bayshore Drive had itself been a dream."

Thorne Shipley remembers that same storm as he and his wife were guests of the Nortons. "During the storm's fury on Miami, we parked our car in the front (of the Nortons) and the hurricane hit . . . and the following morning all the cars were pitted by sand blown up from the beach. They had to be repainted and the windows replaced because the sand was blown so hard.

"Ed Dunlap had given Ed an owl because the anatomy of the owl's eye had not been studied. It was in the freezer and with the power out because of the storm it had to be gotten rid of before it rotted. Ed asked us to take it with us to Key Biscayne to dispose of, but because of the wind it kept coming back at us. Finally a gust took it north and we never saw it again."

In 1963, the entire family, including Patty, the youngest of the children (born May 19, 1961), went to Europe for two months. This vacation was special for several reasons. It was the longest vacation the whole family ever took together. And the famous red and white Volkswagon bus was purchased to provide the family's transportation.

Mary was the dynamo social director who made it happen. They went by ship to Amsterdam, then off to visits in West Germany — to Essen, Dusseldorf, and Giessen in the bus. Happy memories of it abound for all the Norton children, with pauses at the watering holes of Bohemia where some family members "went native."

Reservations ahead were not even thought of. They would detract from the sense of daily adventure that was very much a part of the trip. Carol Ann composed a little ditty about the nightly search for lodgings, and Mary would lead the family in singing it as they bounced along the roads of northern Europe in that most egalitarian family touring car, the Volkswagon bus.

> *Pray to the Lord for an empty Fremdenzimmer*
> *Pray very hard, the light is getting dimmer.*
> *Pray to the Lord that the next one we go by*
> *Might be "Frei."*
> *For we've tried the Tourist Lagen*
> *and we've tried the Volkswagen,*
> *But a gasthaus fremdenzimmer is for me!*

The Wetzig family accompanied them for part of the tour. They remember Ed Norton as tour guide, arising earlier than the rest, walking the streets, talking to the local people in what passed for the native tongue (he could always make himself understood), defining the plan of the day—the sights to be seen and not the

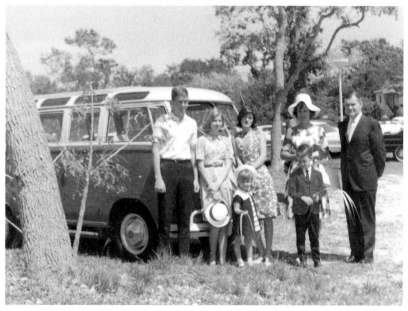

THE VW VAN MIT FAMILIE NORTON

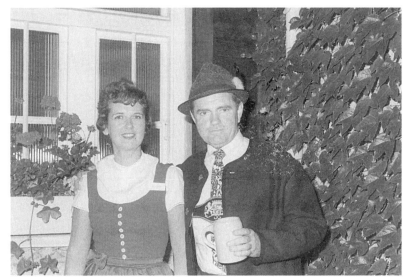

EDWN AND MARY IN LOCAL COSTUME

usual ones that the tourists see, but the offbeat ones that those trained to look beneath the surface would find. All were his self-assigned tasks in which he reveled.

The sojourn in Europe was well deserved for the 41-year-old Ed and 37-year-old Mary. Ed, especially, needed a respite from the demanding pursuit of his dream, which had begun to find concrete realization.

The family was settled in their new home at 2121 South Bayshore Drive, the department was independent, the first of the clinical faculty was recruited, and among prospective resident applicants the department was developing a growing reputation as an excellent teaching program. Here was the beginning of an enormous outpouring of new knowledge. To use a metaphor he often employed, he had tended his grape arbor well and it was now about to bear fruit.

The children adapted to life in South Florida as if they had lived all their lives there. Carol Ann and Marybeth attended Everglades School for Girls. Brian went to Ransom, an elite Coconut Grove school for boys. Kevin and Patti went to Silver Bluff Elementary.

The grandparents Knesnik moved from Yonkers to Coconut Grove in 1964 after Grandpa Knesnik's retirement. Grandpa Emil, an accomplished woodworker renovated the "carriage house" on the property. Ed took as always a keen delight in following the progress of the work. Grandpa Norton and Aunt Helene snowbirded it during the winter months.

All in all, life was a joy for the entire extended family. We were on a journey we weren't sure where to, but we trusted our jovial captain to get us there.

CHAPTER 10

BPEI Grows Like Topsy

1966 – 1972

ALTHOUGH IT WASN'T AT ALL CLEAR AT THE TIME, THE BPEI HAD reached a critical mass of people, energetic faculty, top grade residents, fellows in the subspecialty areas of Ophthalmology — all that was needed to promote growth beyond the expectations of even the architect himself.

Among the fellows, a young German, sensing an opportunity for growth in his specialty area, arrived on BPEI's doorstep. Robert Machemer came in 1966 as a research fellow in the differential radioactive amino acid labeling of retinal cells, but quickly found room for expansion of his fertile imagination, especially with the support of Edward Norton, who understood his work.

Thus began the story of vitreous surgery in Miami. That single development, depending as it did on the happy coincidence of Machemer's insight and the ingenuity of Jean Marie Parel, a Swiss trained engineer and expatriate who joined the faculty from Australia, would have been enough to mark the Bascom Palmer's contribution to American ophthalmology as major. And yet in parallel, Ed Norton, Victor Curtin and Don Gass were beginning to explore in exquisite detail the retina in health and disease with fluorescein angiography and the Zeiss fundus camera, the new tool brought to Miami for completely other purposes by Noble David and Johnny Justice.

Such is the subtle operation of serendipity, of pure chance, alongside the rigor and skepticism of science in the right environment with the right minds there to exploit it.

Don Gass' name is today associated with so many careful studies of the morphology and pathogenesis of retinal diseases that one wonders, what was the rest of Ophthalmology doing between Theodore Leber in the 19th and Don in the 20th century?

Using those same tools, the fundus camera and fluorescein angiography—and the skills of Johnny Justice, a group of clinicians, among them Guy O'Grady and Salvatore Cantolino (pediatrics' first fellow), began to probe the development of retrolental fibro-plasia (as it was then called), a blinding retinal disease of premature infants long held to be conquered by restriction of oxygen.

Thus was a career path fashioned for John Flynn. Though unplanned, he was rewarded in recent decades by seeing that devastating disease now treatable, and blindness prevented by the efforts of many clinicians worldwide.

Doug Anderson, quiet and reserved in his ways, arrived next to begin his contribution to our understanding of glaucoma. His persona was the antithesis of the usual faculty member, who held his views and strongly presented them. This led at times to the raucous discussion, debate and argument that became so characteristic of the Bascom Palmer discourse (unlike the gamesmanship, roundsmanship and one-upsmanship that are the rule at other prestigious institutions).

When Doug spoke ever so carefully and quietly, everybody listened. Discussion, at grand rounds or fluorescein conference for instance, was always within bounds, always seeking truth and clarity of thought — and always presided over by the genial and wise moderator, the Chief, as he was coming to be known, ready with a key question to point out a flaw in one's argument and add a quip or two to soften the blow.

Community ophthalmologists led by Ralph Kirsch, Ken Whitmer, Bob Welsh, Norman Jaffee, Felix DeLaVega, Alfred Smith, and many others were actively encouraged to attend and participate, and they did.

Patients were eager to come to the grand rounds to have their problems presented and discussed, even if the outcome was simply "everything that can be done is being done." They seemed to be aware instinctively they were being seen by the brightest minds in American ophthalmology.

The institution, because of the foresight of its leader, reached out to other centers to train its young in subspecialty areas, something other older established institutions failed to do, to their peril in the fast developing fields of subspecialty ophthalmology.

JLS, as he was known by now, was swamped, primarily due to his "underwater, scuba diving with fins" workup of patients, so christened by the master himself. Part showman (vaudevillian in its best sense), part genius, part pied piper in his ability to attract young medical students and mesmerize them with his antics, he needed help.

A second generation of ophthalmologists was arriving on the scene to fill the ranks of the few (remarkably few) faculty members who had to depart — always sadly, always leaving what they knew was an irreplaceable educational experience, never to be replicated elsewhere.

Bob Sexton in external disease, one of Ed's first recruits, left, and Dick Forster, an early BPEI resident, who had taken a fellowship with Max Fine at the Procter Foundation in San Francisco, returned to take his place.

Joel Glaser (the lineal descendent from Frank Walsh to Lawton, Ed Norton, and Nobby David), returned from training with Bill Hoyt at UCSF with a stop along the way at Queens Square, London, began the training of the third generation of American neuro-ophthalmologists, many of whom bear the stamp of BPEI and some even the phrases, voice and mannerisms of Smith and Glaser. It is

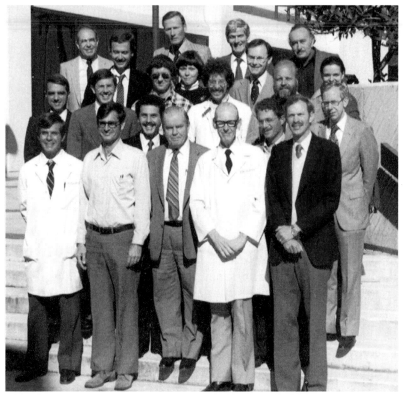

ED NORTON AND HIS FIRST AND SECOND GENERATION FACULTY

not overstating the case to say that there are hundreds of American ophthalmologists who were first turned on to the specialty by these two men.

> *This free-wheeling, unencumbered, joyful and vigorous culture, which took root in Miami and made learning there the experience of a lifetime as it is today, was so described by many of its graduates. And it worked both ways to the benefit of all.*

Alan Byrd, with his wife Sarah and their two boys, came from Moorfields, in London, (as did others later) to study neuro-ophthalmology with Lawton. While in Miami, he became enveloped in the loving embrace of the family Norton as well as the Institute, and he became convinced that the study of the retina, the queen of the sense organs, was his life's calling. So began Alan's illustrious career at the Institute of Ophthalmology and Moorfields.

Sarah Byrd and Mary Norton became closest of friends. Of all the wives of faculty, fellows and residents (for it was still a male dominated culture) Mary and Sarah were probably closest to each other, kindred spirits in outlook. The many pleasant hours they spent together at the pool with the children playing nearby remain a precious memory to Sarah to this day.

With all this growth, happy though it may seem, there had to be a downside. In 1964, Lyndon Johnson, successor to the slain John F. Kennedy, succeeded in getting through a reluctant Congress the Medicare Act of 1965 for coverage of the over-65 age group of Americans. Concessions had to be made, and deals struck with Wilbur Mills, the powerful chairman of the House Ways and Means Committee, and Russell Long (Huey's brother), chairman of the Senate's finance committee.

The two legislative bodies were heavily lobbied against its passage by the then powerful AMA and American College of Surgeons. In their fevered rhetoric it was portrayed by these two institutions as the road to socialism, if not bolshevism.

Whatever this government entitlement program turned out to be or to become (as it is still in process), it was not the road to socialism. For the first time physicians were reimbursed for care that they formerly gave freely as part of the price and privilege of being a physician. An unsubtle change occurred in the ethic of medicine and for the first time a shift from the Brandeis definition of a physician as valuing service above reward became palpable.

The iron law of unintended consequences came into

play here. For a burgeoning academic institution like BPEI with a youthful, busy, and growing faculty, and a resident service facing an annual growth rate of five to seven percent in patient visits, both ensnared in a large 1,200 bed county hospital and more deadly in a county bureaucratic mindset best described as the human equivalent of absolute entropy — at which point in the physical world all motion ceases — this situation set an iron limit on growth.

Faced with the opportunity to fill beds, for which they were reimbursed over long periods of hospitalization for illnesses such as stroke and fractures, combined with the problem of finding beds in nursing homes for indigent patients . . . who had suddenly become private patients by legislative fiat. They chose to fill the beds. There was no recognition, probably no cognition, of growth or productivity.

Opportunity for expansion in operating rooms, or OR time, or growth in any direction was foreclosed. The crush of out-patients in the (by then) outgrown "old" building led to the stopgap purchase of two mobile home trailers, which were connected and outfitted as examining rooms and placed in the parking lot adjacent to the building. This led inevitably to an underhanded and hilarious competition for space, any space, in the trailer in which to examine one's patients. Space was at an absolute premium.

Mrs. Celestine Doty, the prim and gentle woman who was receptionist at the first floor entrance of the BPEI, took pity on the hapless pediatric ophthalmologist then residing on the second floor, jammed with clinic patients to the extent that prisoners from ward D (the county jail) and comatose stroke patients took their place next to the children in the corner designated euphemistically the "waiting room." She would surreptitiously watch when Dr. Norton or Curtin or Gass was at lunch (which wasn't often, by the way), and I could sneak down to see my patients in somewhat more congenial (but by no means luxurious) surroundings.

A nursing service decision to reduce the already paper-thin

operating time because of a shortage of nurses led Victor Curtin, himself a paragon of New England rectitude, to entertain the radical notion that BPEI free itself of that particular tyranny and hire its own nurses to staff the OR. And recruit and hire he did.

Fortunately, Tui Uffenorde, the Jackson-trained head nurse, instead of remaining steadfast to her Jackson nurse sisterhood, threw in her lot with the eye doctors and accompanied them on the journey into a whole new world — the conception, planning, birth, growth and development of a combined eye institute and community eye hospital unlike any other on this continent, nested in an academic setting yet free of many of the toils of that institution.

It was to be a simply breathtaking journey not without risk for

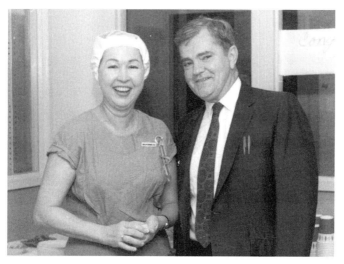

EWDN AND TUI UFFENORDE

all who chose to embark on it. And the people who surrounded Ed Norton now, for the first time, began to sense the journey they were on.

Where some might see crisis and react with withdrawal from its challenge with bitterness, finger pointing and hand wringing, we knew by now that this man would see opportunity, stunning opportunity to attempt something that would be unique in the latter half of the twentieth century.

He would create an academic eye hospital whose staff was open to qualified community ophthalmologists—an institute with a research arm to delve on the deepest level possible into the reasons for, and hopefully the prevention of, the scourge of blindness. It would be comprised of an outpatient clinic and bona fide research facilities. It would remain closely linked to the university, yet financially independent enough to avoid the clutches of that intrusive bureaucracy.

> *A paradox may be understood as something that, while appearing contradictory on its surface, is true and consistent when viewed in the proper light and from the proper perspective.*
>
> *Without Medicare there probably would have been no bed crisis, no nurse crisis. Without Medicare there probably would not have been the sudden privatization of a whole huge demographic slice of American patients over sixty-five years in age, the care of whom, with its consequent revenue stream, would provide the monies necessary to make the dream not only possible but practical.*

And so the first tentative steps, hardly recognizable as such for what they were to portend, were taken in the closing years of the sixties. The retina and cornea service pulled part of their surgery out of Jackson and began to utilize the sadly under-utilized ORs and beds of Highland Park Hospital. Although nominally a small general hospital, Highland Park was almost exclusively a psychiatric in-patient facility with seventeen medical beds and two operating rooms. BPEI took it over—staffing, beds, nurses, orderlies, equipment, supplies — like a starving man devours his first meal.

There was a turbulence to the life of our country during this time. After a "quiet decade" (was it really that?) called, for want of a better appellation the Eisenhower Years, the country entered the sixties with a new president who called on all of us "to do for our country" and not ask from it. It was a rhetorical flourish that touched his listeners' hearts. John Kennedy, the first president to be born in the twentieth century, Irish Catholic, scion of the Kennedy family, seemed to radiate a confidence, a renewal, a vigor, a spirit that had seemed missing somehow in our national life. And Jackie on his arm brought a charm and glamour that melted even the stiff neck and back of Charles De Gaulle of *"La France, c'est moi"* fame.

Alas, it did not last. A disastrous invasion of Cuba, the bungled handiwork of a CIA thoroughly over-intoxicated with its war game playing, was followed soon thereafter by an equally disastrous move on the international chessboard by Nikita Kruschchev to put nuclear weapons in Cuba. The world seemed for an instant to teeter on the brink of the unthinkable.

Scarcely a year later we watched in horror as the young president was cut down at Dealey Plaza in Dallas. And the world seemed to turn upside down for so many. Particularly the young. The old verities no longer sufficed, nor did they believe in them. If Kennedy could be killed so wantonly, was anyone over thirty to be trusted?

Timothy Leary called for a generation to "turn on, tune in, drop out." And they did. They rebelled against their elders. Jerry Rubin and Tom Hayden and Mark Rudd, names that suddenly surfaced as leading this "revolution" of sorts, became instant pop heroes. Their acolytes smoked pot and drank alcohol in its many guises and made love. They were the flower children and Woodstock and Haight-Ashbury became their shrines.

This spirit, so alien to the buttoned-down generation that preceded it, at first was a source of wonder to their elders, then disbelief, and finally, as the tide of events rolled on, of alarm at their young.

Events assumed an ever more chaotic pattern bordering on

generational strife, and names like Viet Nam and Kent State and Watergate were burned into the nation's consciousness and conscience. To this day they remain, just under the surface of our complacent consumer culture waiting to be dredged to the surface again to awaken the bitterest of memories on both sides of the divide.

—

These events touched the lives of a very private Norton family whose three older children were just entering that demi-monde between adolescence and adulthood. At the same time, another heartbreak was in the offing. Its origins go back much further than the sixties.

Sometime during the New York Hospital days, Ed noted pigmentary changes in Mary's retinas. She was without symptoms. Carol Ann remembers being examined and found to have "unusual colorations" in her retinas as well. Thereafter, all five children began to be examined and tested by their father on a regular basis. They called these exams "torture tests." Ed examined the extended Knesnik family as well but found no trace of the problem (except for a brother of Emil who died before testing could be completed).

Later, in Miami, Brian showed some changes similar to his mother's. (He had had an accident one summer in the VW bus, unaware of the approach of another auto from the side; perhaps it was due to loss of peripheral vision.) It was around that time that the first vague suspicion arose of what the condition was — retinitis pigmentosa.

It is not clear if Ed and Mary confided in their son what their suspicions were. They may have decided it best to spare him until he became aware of his loss of night vision and visual field.

Brian was a highly successful scholar at Ransom, and he easily made Harvard, at which time his dad gave him a big hug, perhaps remembering his own difficulties of thirty years before. He excelled in the humanities, history, economics and political science. His bent seemed to be toward the law as a profession, and not medicine. His sisters recall many conversations between father and son about his eyesight and the necessity to take it into account in making career decisions.

Brian and his high school sweetheart Robin Bitter, the daughter of the Dean of UM School of Music, became engaged and married in 1968. Mary and Ed had their first grandchild, Michael John Norton in 1969, a great joy to both of them.

During this period, for reasons not clear, there began a distancing between father and son. Perhaps it was his disease now becoming more manifest and the recognition of its full consequences. Perhaps it was a manifestation of the "son of a famous father" syndrome. Let us subsume them under the title "my father was never there when I needed him." Or, as my own son Thomas (a contemporary of Kevin's) expressed it at a recent Residents Day meeting at BPEI, "You residents were (my father's) sons and I hated you at the time for it."

Should Ed have told him sooner or more fully? How can one judge? The father bore the son's pain, and he did everything in his power to help Brian accept and adapt to his disability through the years. Brian has struggled to come to terms with his father's memory and find peace. In spite of the misunderstandings that led to the flawed bond between Ed and Brian, the love was there. It just never found the right words.

The bitter irony is almost unbearable. Here was arguably the premier retina specialist of his day completely unable to help his first-born son. And he more than anyone else carried the full knowledge of its meaning for him and his future life.

As part of his efforts on behalf of his son, as well as all patients affected with RP, Ed recruited Sam Jacobson, MD, probably BPEI's only true scientist-clinician (with the emphasis on "scientist"). Sam has devoted his professional life to the study of RP and has made very significant contributions to our understanding.

Sam described his relationship with Ed: "Before my job interview with Dr. Norton in 1983, I was told by others that if EWDN believed it was time to start research in hereditary retinal degenerations, he will do so. And, if it was not time, nothing that I could say would convince him. As I sat at the long table to the right of Dr. Norton in his McKnight office and watched him make notes on his yellow legal pad, I recognized that he felt it was definitely the time for Bascom Palmer Eye Institute to start research into these incurable forms of blindness. He offered the job; I was honored and promptly accepted.

"After a handshake, he set the direction for my career with the words, 'Sam, I expect you to create a retinal degeneration research center second to none in the world.' I am still trying to live up to the goals he set for me. I think he would forgive me for not yet having a cure, and I know he would be proud of the progress this field has made since 1983."

Kevin, the second son, was also experiencing the wave of rebellion sweeping across this nation. His school, Ransom, bore the brunt of Kevin's rebellion or at least its new headmaster did. Ed and Mary sent Kevin on a sabbatical senior year to Israel, where he met and later married his first wife, Renee Rachow.

The path of rebellion that marked his generation continued well into his emergence into adult life. Carol Ann, Mary Beth and Patty seemed to carry on with their lives although they were very aware and sensitive to the family difficulties.

Carol Ann, two years older than Brian, went to Wellesley and overlapped with him at Harvard during her last two years. After graduation she worked for a time in Washington and, in 1970, married her high school sweetheart, Neilsen Rogers, who was in the US Navy. After a sojourn on overseas duty in Italy (the armed services had relented on that prohibition by then), they moved to San Francisco, where a second grandchild, Jennifer, was born in 1973.

Mary Beth followed her father and brother to Harvard. Patti, the youngest child, was the last one at home with Mary and Ed.

The decade of the seventies was marked by the loss of loved ones. Jackie, Ed's brother, died on May 18, 1976. Gentle, quiet and reserved, Jackie was a frequent guest of the Nortons. At these times he took the opportunity to attend sports and school activities of the Norton children. His sudden and unexpected death was a particular shock to Ed and his father because Jackie was always more robust than Ed.

Grandpa Knesnik died in 1974, Grandma Knesnik in 1978 and Grandpa Norton in 1977. These grandparents were very close and dear to the Norton children. The losses added a note of sadness to the family life in what was often referred to as the "Golden Years" of Ed Norton's Bascom Palmer.

CHAPTER 11

BPEI/ABLEH: The Dream Is Born

1972 – 1976

FRED COWELL, FAR AND AWAY THE BEST OF THE JACKSON HOSPITAL administrators with whom Norton dealt during his tenure, was acutely aware of the dilemma faced by Ophthalmology, a dilemma caused by the accident of its own success. Fred, a "thinking man's administrator" (as well as a tennis partner of Ed's), was a hard but fair bargainer when it came time to negotiate the "AOA" or Annual Operating Agreement between Jackson Hospital (representing Dade County) and Bascom Palmer.

This agreement defined the reimbursement that the county would pay BPEI for the care of the county's indigent patients. It was manifestly one-sided and unfair: the indigent patients received care from the best eye faculty in the country and the Institute was reimbursed a pittance for that care. Cowell was probably more aware of the problem than any of the others on his side of the table.

In response to what was becoming an intolerable situation, Dade did what one would expect any "cover my *derriere*" bureaucracy to do. It appointed a committee to come up with a "plan." Fortunately, at the very moment that plan seemed to turn serious (it was never to be completed), another arm of the county purchased the land across the street from Bascom Palmer and the property became available for lease.

Don Gass immediately recognized this as an answer to a major problem. They should build a new Bascom Palmer, and this was the ideal location. The opportunity it offered — to build a completely new facility from the ground up — in the sheer avoidance of a myriad of problems of governance, finance, architecture and staff-

118

ing was breathtaking. As well as providing generous space to expand the physical facilities of the institute to grow into, it promised something much more precious: autonomy.

No one saw this more clearly than Ed Norton and he immediately seized the property, tying it up in a ninety-nine-year lease from the county. All his career up to now had pointed to such an opportunity. Each step he had taken seemed to prepare him for this moment. He was ready. He had trained himself as a physician and teacher, sharpened his wit as a negotiator and businessman, honed his skills as a fund raiser and an administrator. Nestled among those talents, hidden from view up to now, was the talent of the artist and architect, now about to become manifest in the realization of the dream.

At this point, Ed Norton's life and the dream and its realization became fused. There is no doubt in the author's mind that without his commitment of will from the outset, BPEI/ABLEH would never have happened. It brought the man enormous gratification to see it grow from an idea into a practical reality. It brought him accolades from his colleagues that embarrassed him. It gave him the simple pleasure of a task spectacularly well done against many, many obstacles. It brought new challenges to his many-faceted intellect which, in meeting them, gave him delight.

It also brought him more separation from his faculty and his residents and fellows, as well as from his family; because of the institution's ravenous demands he could no longer be with any of them as closely as he had before. There were simply too many things to do, too many administrative duties to attend to. We all credited it to the simplistic phrase, "We're getting too big." Too big for what?

He was, according to the by-laws of the hospital, its medical director. As chairman of the department he continued to bear the responsibility for the education of eighteen residents and twenty-odd post-residency fellows.

The task the man had shouldered forced him to become his own de facto administrator and comptroller, though he had, in a feat of patient argumentation and persuasion, won from the county and the university the approval and autonomy, *mirabile dictu*, to select a hospital administrative firm, HCA (Hospital Corporation of America) to perform these functions.

Norton was his own fund-raiser *par excellence* and worked at that with the same intensity he gave all the other pursuits, and with a success that bordered on the miraculous. He used to say "people give to people," and if that be true, then the benefactors of the two institutions (BPEI and ABLEH) must have valued him immensely.

The full details of the hospital building are in Victor Curtin's Edward Norton Lecture delivered to the Miami Ophthalmological Society on 2/26/96. (The text is obtainable by contacting Doris Silver, archivist, the Mary and Edward Norton Library, BPEI.) The concept called for a one-hundred-bed eye hospital with six operating rooms, and clinic spaces on the lower floors to accommodate sixty-four examining rooms and a core of ancillary services.

Architectural plans called originally for a five-story building of 190,000 square feet with an option to include two shell floors. Total cost estimated at $6,500,000. Mrs. Anne Bates Leach of Palm Beach, a strong supporter of Ed Norton, as was her husband, convinced her friend Mrs. Celeste Sanford, also of that city, to contribute $1,300,000. The building was named for Mrs. Leach.

When the plans were submitted for bids, the low bid was $9,500,000. A shock, to say the least. To raise the required amount, a tax exempt hospital construction bond issue under the Tax Exempt Health Care Facility status of Dade County was approved by both the board of commissioners of Dade and the board of trustees of the university.

The financial validity of the bond issue was evaluated by Moody's, a Wall Street firm, given an AAA rating, the safest possible,

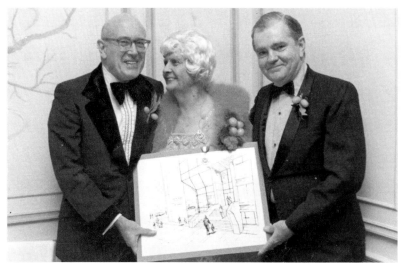

EWDN, HENRY KING STANFORD, AND ANNE BATES LEACH

and sold out within forty-five minutes of the offering. Significant in the bond prospectus is the statement that their redemption, both interest and principle, *was the responsibility of the Bascom Palmer faculty.*

Ground was broken for the new building in April 1973. As Victor Curtin says in his Norton Lecture, "The estimated completion time was eighteen months—a monumental understatement." The seven-story building was completed and opened thirty-nine months later, on July 5, 1976.

VTC was credited by his admirers (the author among them), with magical powers of discernment. It has proven a useful rule of thumb to apply the "Curtin rule" to any prediction of construction completion (of anything from a bird bath to a commercial building): take the builder's estimate, double it, and add three units of the estimate (months, years, whatever), and that will be about right.

At the groundbreaking ceremony was Jack Norton, Ed's dad; this is one of the few photos we have of the two men together.

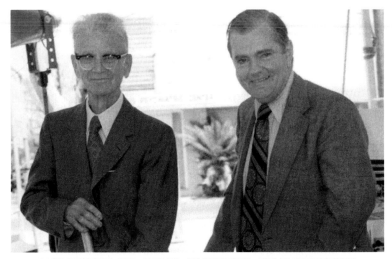

JACK NORTON AND SON ED AT HOSPITAL GROUNDBREAKING

Ed Norton loved a good party, and one of the best the BPEI ever hosted was the combined celebration of the nation's bicentennial and the opening of the new edifice. Ed's friends and admirers and friends of the faculty came from all over. Luminaries from the world of ophthalmology studded the program. Lay leaders, academic dignitaries, his own family and friends, residents, ex-residents, fellows and families, politicians from the Dade county and the Miami political establishment (always anxious to appear at any event that would display them in the kindest possible light), the wealthy people and the simple people that so entranced him. It was a wonderful and exhilarating experience for everyone and a treasured memory for those privileged to participate.

The aesthetic aspects of the building were the work of the architectural firm of Candela and Spillas; the functional aspects the work of the faculty. It was a labor of love for all of us and everybody on the faculty contributed ideas.

Ed Norton and the author contributed the major impulse for the pod design of the outpatient spaces — the doctors inside the pod were free to move from exam room to exam room away from the anxious entreaties of the waiting patients. Victor Curtin and Gaby Kressly, the "Departmental Dragon" as she is affectionately known to some of her admirers, designed a unique hospital room that could be easily converted to a motel room. The design even incorporated a small self-serve kitchen on the northwest corner of the fifth floor, where meals could be prepared and eaten cafeteria-style by the patient and family.

> *When the building was planned, the average length of stay was five days for a cataract and seven to ten days for a retinal detachment operation. The room design embodied the notion that eye patients typically required skilled nursing care for the first day or so but thereafter could be cared for by a family member who could live in and provide every-thing needed.*

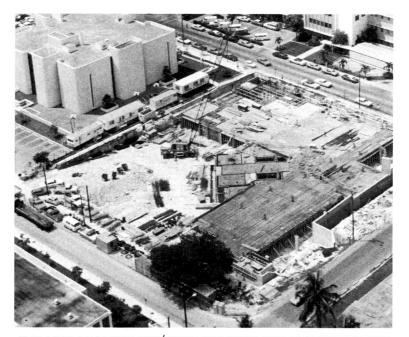

THE LAND ON WHICH BPEI/ABLEH WAS BUILT. THE FOOTPRINT OF THE BUILDING'S "L" SHAPE CAN CLEARLY BE SEEN IN THE GROUND FLOOR.

It was for its time an advanced notion, only to be superceded in a few years by the revolution that swept Ophthalmology into its future as an out- patient surgical specialty.

Redoubtable Tui Uffenorde ("Uffie" to her surgeon charges) and Robert Machemer designed the operating rooms. Each room was a gem, fully equipped with overhead microscope, a novel-design OR table that was in fact the patient's hospital bed (to save the awkward and at times backache-inducing transfer of patient to and from the stretcher), TV monitors to video the surgery, foot pedals to control the XYZ axes and focus of the scope — they had the latest state of the art in every detail.

Every feature of the building was examined under the obsessive detail-oriented minds of the many ophthalmologists involved. And more than anyone else, Ed Norton recognized tiny design flaws and inconsistencies that forever secured his reputation as a builder and planner. It left all of us around the table awestruck at his skill. And it wasn't just in picking nits that he excelled; it was that he

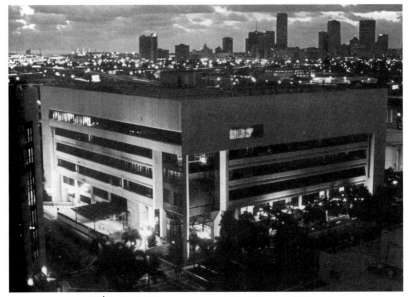

BPEI/ABLEH AT SUNSET. THE DREAM COME TRUE.

had a computer graphics mind before the software was invented.

Still, in spite of all our efforts, there were two major design flaws in the building. One had a hilarious outcome; the other not so hilarious. The first concerns the dimensions of the central staircase. The archetects, who were novices in planning a hospital, designed a staircase of the dimensions used for a commercial building. Several inspectors passed it with flying colors but the state fire marshal inspector, to the best of my recollection, found that the stairway was too narrow for a hospital and refused to certify the building. What to do?

The building was well along in construction, and the required change called for a major redesign of the central core. This was done and the stairway enlarged to be large enough to accommodate abreast the Red Army or the Peoples Army of the Republic of China had they needed to ascend or descend it for any reason. At least that little jibe served to add a humorous touch to the costly and time-consuming flaw.

The second problem was the placement of the library. It is, in its ground floor location, precariously close to the level of the water table. Despite skepticism from both Ed Norton and Victor Curtin, the architects insisted that water-tight construction of that segment of the building was possible. When the South Florida rains came in Biblical deluge proportion, as they do from time to time, they flooded portions of that lowest floor.

Today this space is the Mary and Edward Norton Library, a tribute to both of them from grateful alumni and faculty who had the good sense to get the endowment raised while Ed still lived. It was the most fitting gift his students could give him. After his retirement the library provided him with many hours of pleasure, sitting in the rare book room, reading from the treasured works of the past that he had acquired over a lifetime of collecting.

Ed, as William Osler, was a dedicated philologist. Now he had

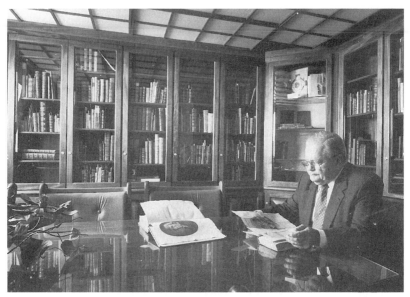

ED NORTON IN THE KIRSCH RARE BOOK ROOM

time to read those treasures and share some of the wisdom in their pages with anyone nearby, primarily Reva Hurtes, the librarian from its inception and one of the "glue girls."

> *This is a term of affection and respect, my own name for the women who formed the matrix of dedicated service and loyalty to the institution and any and all who sought its help — former residents, fellows, patients, students, physicians from elsewhere, and ordinary people seeking help of any kind that was so much a part of what BPEI came to mean throughout the world. They included Celestine Doty, Gaby Kressly, Jean Newland, Patsy Carnahan, Marie Guanci, Pearl Goldberg, Betsy Barton, Kathy Barton Corser (the only mother-daughter team as far as I know), Margaret Bertolame, and Mary Jeanne Williams.*

A final word about the library. Its shelves contain one of the finest collections of books, journals, and periodicals as well as rare incunabula of the eye and visual system in the world, housed in a structure, with paneling and shelves and walls that give it a warmth and beauty that strike the eye of the beholder, inviting him or her to rest here, to study and to learn.

Again the touch of Norton. He had come across the work of

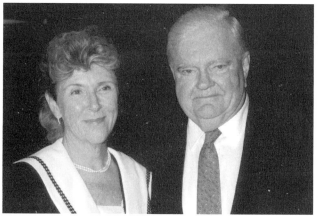

EWDN AND REVA HURTES

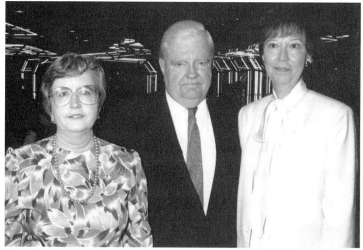

EWDN WITH GABY KRESSLY AND YVONNE KARRENBERG

two struggling wood craftsmen-artists in Coral Gables—Bill Frohbose (deceased) and Randy Beers—and recognized the beauty and talent of their work. With the library he gave the two their first big contract, and (as with Peter Jefferson, the architect of his home) their careers took off.

As Randy Beers tells it: "It was in 1980 at a reception in Coconut Grove that my partner and I first met Dr. Ed Norton. Some of our handcrafted wood creations were on display for the event. Dr. Norton decided then and there that he would trust two unknown woodworkers and artists to create the Honduras mahogany library, study area, card catalogues and rare book room for the world-renowned Bascom Palmer Eye Institute in Miami. He gave us our first big break.

"We had to expand our operations and hire more cabinetmakers just to handle this huge project. It has been our honor to complete many other projects for Dr. Norton over the years, one of which was his personal desk. That was over twenty-one years ago, and thanks to Dr. Norton's trust and belief we are still creating with the integrity and craftsmanship valued by Dr. Norton."

In my den is the table from Ed's office, the scene of so many memorable and unmemorable faculty meetings presided over by the Chief. It was lovingly remodeled to fit the smaller space by these same two craftsmen, who were delighted with the opportunity to pay a last tribute to his memory. It is one of the treasures of my BPEI years. And it is about as full and messy as it was when he kept his many projects on it. All of us have these — some tangible, some only memories. Each brightens our lives in its own way.

CHAPTER 12

BPEI/ABLEH: Growing Pains

1976 – 1985

As Victor Curtin says, for a building that has had so many dedications, it is entirely right and proper that it have a baptism. In November, 1976, the water main serving the high pressure sprinkler system burst. Water dissected the soil outside the library and flooded the tiled moat surrounding the ground floor below street level. The glass panes held fast and the library and photography— priceless and irreplaceable assets of the BPEI—were both saved.

This test, which passed with flying colors in '76, augured well for the future, as the structure was to be sorely tested again by hurricane Andrew in 1992, which it again passed without major damage and actually served as a temporary home for many whose homes were demolished in that storm.

The new BPEI/ABLEH opened to see outpatients on July 5, 1976. The first surgical procedure was done by George Blankenship, MD, on September 5, the day after Labor Day. George was one of the second generation of faculty. Famous for his wry sense of humor and ebullience, George would, during his years at BPEI, enliven many a Saturday morning faculty meeting with his irreverent quips.

Those first years of operation were somewhat anxious ones financially. The hospital was built as a community eye hospital. Where was the community?

Although there existed literally no town-gown conflict of any dimension, thanks largely to the policy begun by Norton of operating strictly as a tertiary care faculty and practice — you had to have a referral from an ophthalmologist to be seen at BPEI — the community ophthalmologists soon found that some of their patients did not like the thought of coming downtown to an unknown place to have their eye surgery. In addition, the community hospitals did not universally applaud their ophthalmological staff departing to a competing facility, even if there was no comparison in professional staffing, equipment and safety for the patients.

After all, these were the heady days when ophthalmologists, with their quick turnover and high reimbursement rate, were the darlings of the bottom line in those hospitals. A far cry from today when Ophthalmology is a poor relation on any hospital spreadsheet and a loss leader.

With time and the dawning recognition of just how good the nursing care provided by Judy Tashjian, RN (another of the glue girls) and Uffi's staff in the OR, the patients came, a trickle at first, then a steady stream, a river and then such a torrent that four new ORs had to be built (adding to the existing six) to handle the tide.

The battle over control of the institution, having been fought and won, the hospital was easily the busiest and most impressive in size and numbers on the medical school campus. It remained to be demonstrated to that skeptical and frustrated bureaucracy, Dade County and the nervous and vacillating university Board of Trustees, that the marriage of a private sector management firm and an imaginative CEO (and CFO and medical director all in one) could work. And work it did!

Those early years were ones of growth for the structure that had been built seemingly far in excess of its needs. It almost overwhelmed us by its dimensions. But thus were the workings of Ed Norton's mind. He planned far ahead of today, at times beyond tomorrow's horizon.

The residency was growing both in quality and quantity. From three residents per year in the sixties to four and then five in the seventies and six in the eighties, it paralleled the rise in the number of patients, medically indigent by the county's standards, coming to the second floor eye clinic for care. Norton used to joke that if the residents ever wanted to commemorate anybody for the success of their training program, they should raise a statue to *El Maximo Lider*, Fidel Castro, whose machinations in the Caribbean and Latin America resulted in turmoil and a steady tide of refugees (the prototypical clinic patient at BPEI) washed up on the sands of South Florida.

The medical student world, in spite of its wide dispersion over the North American continent, was cohesive in its tight communications network. Word soon spread to the farthest reaches of the continent that there was something magic going on in South Florida that needed at least a look.

If things didn't seem quite right, they could always fall back on those old standbys, Mass. Eye and Ear and Wilmer. These boys (and later girls) learned that not only was it true what their friends from Florida had told them, but it was fun along with the hard work. (Just like their Florida friends said.) By now it was the seventies, and even veterans of the Students for a Democratic Society (SDS) were admitted among the resident classes.

Nobody worked harder or seemed to have more fun than the quiet man in the rumpled Sears Roebuck suit and the Thom McAnn boy scout shoes, as they used to portray him in the end-of-the-year residents day skit. A fashion plate he never was.

Now, however, he was a little thicker about the middle, a little slower in his step, and a little more often gone —"on the road" —because of the heavy demands of leadership that American Ophthalmology thrust upon him. Not because he sought it; he never did. But because all sorts of organizations — from the newly formed National Eye Institute (in the founding of which he played a key role), to the American Board of Ophthalmology (ABO), the oldest of America's boards, responsible to the American public for the quality of the product trained in our residencies, to the American

Academy of Ophthalmology (AAO), undergoing a wrenching separation from the otolaryngologists with whom they had been united
since 1916 — all needed this man.

And his reward? He was the subject of a lawsuit (along with
Melvin Rubin, secretary for instruction, and Bruce Spivey, the
executive vice president of the Academy, and the Academy itself),
asking damages of $34 million for violation of anti-trust laws.
Their crime? The Academy Board had endorsed on behalf of the
Academy the statement of the National Advisory Eye Council that
radial keratotomy was an experimental procedure and its results and
its safety were not established. (The procedure involves cutting the
cornea with four to eight spoke-like incisions to reduce its optical
power, to correct myopia.)

The attack was mounted by some Academy members more
concerned with their immediate pecuniary gain from the refractive
surgery bonanza than the caution that the Academy and Norton as
its president felt the public should be aware of until all the evidence
was in (it still isn't).

That lawsuit was fought institutionally by the Academy and
personally by Norton, Spivey (a close friend of his later years) and
Rubin, who was dropped from the suit before trial. At trial, the jury,
seeing through the sham of the anti-trust "restraint of trade" argument raised by the plaintiffs, found all defendants not guilty on
all counts. In a little-known side issue, all the defendants refused
repeated offers of a "deal" by the plaintiffs, and settle for nominal
damages, preferring instead to go to trial rather than back down on
the issue of whether the warning was prudent and ethical.

Few knew of the struggle or the time it cost or the potential for
ruinous penalties, civil and perhaps criminal, had the parties been
found guilty.

It is appropriate here to recount Edward Norton's role in the
history of the AAO. His early role was as a member of the council
of the Academy, focused on the separation of Ophthalmology from

Otolaryngology, with which they had been joined since 1896. His quiet voice and reasoned, non-confrontational style were appreciated by both sides and helped keep the separation amicable.

David Noonan, who was recruited to be deputy executive vice-president of the AAO, recounts Ed's intervention on his personal behalf: "Ed got me cornered and convinced me there was only one possible selection I could make if I wanted to hitch my wagon to a rising star."

Ed's next task involved the site for the 1980 annual meeting. New Orleans had been selected a decade before. But the Academy had outgrown its San Francisco site in 1979. Mel Rubin, on investigating New Orleans for its suitability for the expanded instruction courses, informed the board that the space available was even more inadequate.

Ed, accompanied by Bruce Spivey and David Noonan, flew to New Orleans and sat down with the New Orleans Visitors Convention Bureau, which had a signed contract. Bruce says of that meeting, "Ed, in his usual unflappable way as the kind of person given a problem, went about solving it."

He pointed out to the convention bureau members how helpful it would be in their negotiations with city fathers to use this withdrawal as evidence of their great need for suitable convention space. Is that a politician or what? In return for a promise to come back at a later date when the facilities were expanded (a promise kept by the Academy), they were released from their contract.

Now they were free to negotiate with Chicago, a much larger venue. The next task was to meet with the convention people in Chicago and negotiate an almost "spur of the moment" deal for only ten months hence — an almost unheard of feat.

Unfortunately, the joy of the Chicago meeting was somewhat dimmed for all of us, as it must have been so much more so for Ed, as Mary had passed away the previous July. His sister Polly and his daughters and sons joined him, however, and that helped him greatly.

Later, Ed traveled to Paris with David Noonan and Bruce Spivey and his wife, Amanda. David recalls the day the group journeyed to Giverney to see Monet's home and famous gardens. Only on this day, a Monday, the site was closed to the public.

Ed, never at a loss for solutions, suggested a trip to the back of the property to see if a peek over the fence was possible. As the group made their way to the back via a narrow alley they encountered a workman fussing with the lock on the back fence. The fluent linguist in Ed Norton rose to the occasion and he implored the workman to let them take a quick walk through the gardens. *Voila!* Five strangers from America had the lily pond and the Japanese bridge and the rest all to themselves!

To return to the theme of these years, the building. The institution, fertile and growing in its faculty and training programs, had in a matter of two decades become an educational resource looked up to by both the world of ophthalmology and the myriad of eye patients seeking the best care they could find. Yet it had no suitable venue to hold its meetings, conferences, seminars and grand rounds.

The structure had two arms extending from two sides of a square. Part of the master plan for the new building had been the concept of completing the square with a triangular-shaped auditorium as the center of the academic and educational activity (not just for the department but for the whole medical campus).

Ground was broken in 1978 for a 200-seat amphitheater, raised to the height of the second floor and connected by a glass-walled walkway to the main building. The construction was overseen in detail by Robert Knighton, PhD, and, wonder of wonders, was completed on schedule. Its largest donors were Edith and Earl Retter, patients of Don Gass; the building was named for them.

Novel seating arrangements proved successful, with so-called "United Nations" seating in the front (though no one has yet taken off his shoe and banged it on the table for attention), and theater seating in its rear ten rows. Its acoustics are superb, thanks to the decision to avoid all the contradictory and confusing advice given by many "experts."

The beautiful Retter Auditorium has been home to many memorable and unique learning experiences. Among the varied uses is as a venue for the Curso Inter Americano, a post-Academy meeting for Latin American ophthalmologists (and shopping expeditions for their wives and families) on their way home from the annual meeting. The meeting was the brainchild of Don Nicholson, one of the second generation BPEI ophthalmologists, who contributed more than anyone to opening Latin America to the Eye Institute and vice versa. (Due to its immense and growing popularity the Curso can no longer be held in the 200-seat Retter, as its annual attendance exceeds three hundred fifty participants.)

Beneath the Retter Auditorium is the Retter Cafe, which was built to supplement the cafeteria in the basement of the BPEI, where

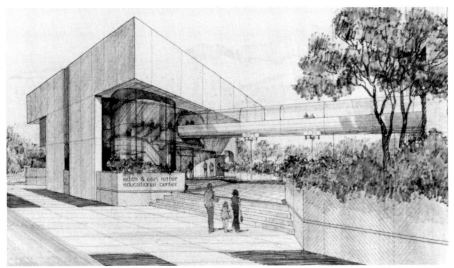

ARTIST'S RENDITION OF THE RETTER AUDITORIUM

space was inadequate to handle all the hungry who wanted to eat there. An awning covered its patio style seating. Although there was strong sentiment among some of the faculty, residents and employees to call it "Ed's Place," which would have been completely appropriate, it was named the Retter Cafe, due to a cooler head (Ed's) that prevailed.

Quality is another touch built into so many aspects of the Institute by Ed Norton. And just as he had found the two craftsmen (Frohbose and Biers) who lent artistry to the Norton Library, he found Steve Chess, caterer extraordinaire, who could add a touch of culinary class to even the simplest snack, something so typically wanting in hospital menus.

Over the years the cafe has become a gathering place for breakfast or lunch for many different groups on the medical campus. Indeed, it became a standing joke that the best attended meeting of all, with the emphasis on all members of the staff, community, residents, and retirees, was the quarterly staff meetings held at 7 AM. Not because of the program by any means—it covered the routine and mundane matters that have to do with the running of the hospital—but simply because the food was so delicious and presented such a variety to please any eye and palate.

During the dedication ceremony of the building there was a moment of sadness for Ed, somehow shared by all who were there. No one can forget the very poignant moment when Ed introduced his family; when he came to Mary's name a quiet sob escaped him. Mary was hospitalized at Mercy Hospital for her continuing depression.

Mary, always the wonderful, giving, spontaneous, caring "parent by proxy" to so many of her husband's faculty, fellows and residents, was, in addition to that almost full-time vocation, an active member of her community. She was a trustee of Everglades School. She was a board member of the Children's Home Society.

Mary gave of herself to all her activities much as her husband did.

Carol Ann recalls a spontaneous family reunion that occurred in 1969. Mary was a delegate to the national convention of the CHS in Philadelphia; there was at the same time an anti-war protest march in Washington, DC. Mary drove down from Philidelphia and stayed with Carol Ann. Brian and Robin and new son Michael drove down from Cambridge, and the family all went to the protest march together with friends.

It has been said that Ed, watching TV at home in Coconut Grove, saw his family protesting the war! It's too good an embellishment to pass up here even if it isn't quite true.

Although Mary never participated in other protests, it was clear where she stood with regard to this conflict, as was true of many Americans by this time. The young had clearly seen how wrong this war was long before their elders could admit it. And oh, how right they were!

> *By that time the official government of the people, by the people and for the people had become so estranged from those very people that Washington evinced a bunker mentality. Official lie piled on official lie as body bags by the thousands quietly came home to warriors' funerals. Government—executive, judicial and legislative—was paralyzed, trapped in a web of deception of its own people and its own making. It took the people, simple people like Mary and her son and daughters, to take to the streets to force the government of the United States of America to reverse its course and extricate itself from the horror it had created.*
>
> *Mary and others like her were true patriots and participants in what was probably the most serious test of American democracy in the twentieth century.*

Kevin tells a beautiful story of his mother's charity, so typical of her. One afternoon, somewhere about this time, he was with her in a Coconut Grove cafe frequented by hippies. She left her purse open at the table with a twenty dollar bill hanging out. One of the patrons sauntered over and took the twenty. He was stopped at the door by other patrons who asked her if they should call the police. Without a pause she opened her purse, took out the rest of the money in it and gave it to the man and said, "If you need more just ask."

Mary was becoming increasingly night blind and increasingly depressed as the RP began to destroy her sight at almost the same time as Brian's. Depressed in a time when we didn't talk much about it, and had still less, pitifully less, to do for it.

Mary walked the whole Calvary of depression and progressive night blindness, but not alone. Ed never left her side, as she had never left his during those long years when she was, in effect, his only supporter and the major parent to five children. Our hearts ached for them both, but in that peculiar way of the Celts nobody spoke a word of their pain. During that period, Ed and Mary drew ever closer. He took, for the first time in memory, Mondays off to have lunch with her, to go to counseling or to a museum or shopping or whatever.

Mary's pain ended on July 23, 1980 when Ed awoke to find his beloved Mary dead beside him in their bed. CPR was of no avail.

Kevin, then living with his wife in the carriage house, recalls his father sitting in their living room as if in a trance. He did the utterly right thing: he called Victor Curtin. Within moments Vic came, took Ed by the arm and walked with him for hours in the park.

Now alone—Mary gone and the children grown and starting their own lives and families—he was alone as he had never been since those lonely hours as a sick child condemned to rest in bed for weeks on end. Eventually feeling returned, and Ed could begin again to pick up his life, so successful to the world outside and so shattered in the world inside, with worn out and broken tools and put it back together again.

For about a year and a half following Mary's death Ed had Sunday dinner with the Curtins, a welcome respite for this most social of men. It was during this time as well that he visited his grandchildren, and solidified his friendships with Pierre Amalric, Bruce Spivey and, of course, Paul Wetzig. Slowly, his life began to take shape again.

It was during this time that Gordon Miller, one of his early residents, introduced him to Charlotte Breyer Rogers. Charlotte was a vivacious and outgoing woman, an heiress to the Breyer Ice Cream fortune, probably known as a socialite in her own circles. She and Ed "hit it off" from the first. They shared a love of travel, good conversation, and good food and drink. She quickly became interested in his life's work and his dreams for its further development.

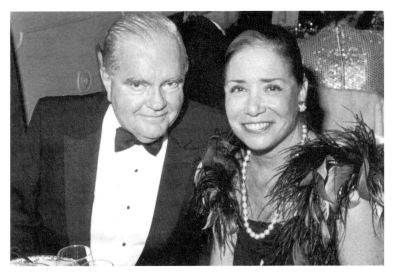

EWDN AND CHARLOTTE BREYER ROGERS

She contributed to the realization of those dreams by endowing the Edward W.D. Norton Chair of Ophthalmology with Ed as its first holder. And when Dade county decided to close the speedway known as Tenth Avenue between BPEI/ABLEH and Jackson's Clinic, she permanently endowed the mall, which was named the "Breyer Patch" in her honor.

Charlotte was Ed's late life friend and confidant. Neither one stood in awe of the other. She was secure in her family heritage and great wealth, he in his great accomplishments and prominence in ophthalmology. They spent a good deal of happy time together from 1983 until the end of her life in November, 1988.

CHAPTER 13

BPEI Matures:
Change Works Its Way

1985 – 1992

ONE WOULD HAVE THOUGHT THAT AFTER THE ORDERED YET hectic growth of the institution in the last decade and a half it was time for its prime mover to rest on his laurels. By now these were broad enough and recognition of his accomplishments was universal. In twenty-five years he had founded Bascom Palmer, carefully selected his faculty and imbued each with a measure of his zeal and dedication, seen his resident classes grow each year in size and quality, and tended the "vines" (as he called his donors) in his "vineyard."

It was time. But it didn't happen. Change forced him to remain flexible, to meet the challenges of today and, because of his ability to see over the horizon to tomorrow, the changes that he saw coming. Having sensed their approach he could no more rest than he could walk away from their challenge.

Ferment was in the air. The whole health care edifice built up so laboriously since the time of the Flexner report (the 1910 survey of medical education in the US commissioned by the Carnegie Foundation) was being questioned as inefficient, wasteful, and far too costly.

The survey indicted the professional training of physicians as little more than a sham, a fast-buck diploma mill racket. It induced a shocked university community to take over the training of physicians in the university-based medical schools. Thus began the gradual ascent of modern American medicine out of the dark ages to the pinnacle it enjoyed in the post WWII era of the biologically-based model of the practice of scientific medicine.

Edward Norton was one of the biological model's most dedicated apostles. Everything he had done professionally could be understood in terms of medicine's relentless drive to push back ignorance and disease to provide, as Macfarlane Burnett, the father of modern immunology and Australia's Nobel Laureate, so succinctly put it, "The true aim of medicine in the broadest sense is to provide for every human being, from conception to death, the greatest fullness of health and length of life that is allowed by their genetic constitution and the accidents of life."

But forces beyond the control of any human (in some sense blessings), chief among them the growth of scientific knowledge and the aging of the population (who now enjoyed decades more of life than their parents and grandparents), were the dynamos driving the rise in health care consumption and its costs.

How did it play out in one small microcosm of the universe, the BPEI? It drove up hospital costs to the point that some community ophthalmologists could no longer freely bring their patients to the institution. The federal government, fully cognizant of what was happening to the Medicare trust fund and able to spin out its actuarial future, began to drastically reduce inpatient cataract reimbursement. For a one-hundred-bed eye hospital this could, unchecked, result in a sheriff appearing at the hospital door, padlocking it, and posting a notice to creditors where to seek payment for their debts. A nightmare scenario.

True to the Darwinian definition of a survivor, Ed Norton literally turned on a dime. He made major and minor changes on the sixth floor of the hospital: he turned it into an outpatient surgical center—well before other eye hospitals in the country did it.

Although little noticed except as a smooth transition, it was long and costly because of that *bete noir*; the state bureaucracy had asserted its primacy and established a whole new set of standards to which the original six ORs and the four new ones had to adhere.

The design of a demi-room or cubicle, where patients

would be prepared for surgery and to which they would return after, to be discharged home that same day, was a feature of the transformation copied by many other hospitals. The state of Florida was first to be forced to change primarily because the community was always in the gunsights of the federals for fraud and abuse of Medicare (taxpayers) dollars. And in this there was some truth, as history has shown.

But from the very inception of Medicare, there was never any question about billing for services not rendered (to Medicare or any third party payor). No absentee charges, no signing of charts without the doctor having seen the patient, no hint of the scandals that later beset the HCA organization, when it became Columbia-HCA, Inc. (They were forced to pay the largest civil penalty in history, some three quarters of a billion dollars in fines for just such hanky panky in other hospitals they owned or managed. Not to mention criminal indictments not yet adjudicated.)

Jean Newland, one of the "glue girls," knowing her boss as she did and responsible to him alone for the fiscal soundness of the department, knew he would never countenance anything but what was absolutely right.

By 1988, the change over to outpatient surgery was undertaken and the north wing with thirty-six hospital beds was converted to a smooth running outpatient surgical center. As Victor Curtin remarked in his Norton Lecture, "I believe we eluded a dedication on this project."

In the mid-sixties another challenge arose from an unexpected quarter. As noted earlier, because of a deficit of funds on hand for the building ($6.5 million) and the low bid ($9.5 million), a tax exempt bond issue of $8.5 million was floated successfully on Wall Street in 1972. The extra dollars were to assure that the sixty-four examining rooms and all the hospital rooms and ancillary spaces could be adequately equipped and ready to go when the building opened on July 5, 1976. Most of the bonds were of twenty years duration—to be redeemed from revenues generated by the Institute. All the bonds would have been redeemed by 1992, a target well within reach by the early 1980s.

Then, without consulting Dr. Norton, without a word of warning to him, the Board of Trustees renegotiated the bond issue. "To obtain a more favorable rate of interest" was the explanation given for the action. In so doing the term of indebtedness was extended from 1992, when the BPEI/ABLEH would have been completely debt-free and without lien of any kind, to 2008.

> *The reason rings hollow when it is realized that the debt will be redeemed by faculty members who had nothing to do with contracting it, and they will, using earnings from operations reimbursed at lower levels than they were in the 1980s. One has only to look at what has happened to the physician fee side of the equation in health care in the last decade to know just how difficult that added burden will be.*

Although the bond prospectus for the new issue placed the "full faith and credit of the University of Miami" behind the redemption, one can't conceive of a penny ever leaving their coffers as long as there is a Bascom Palmer to make the payments. Forgive a confession of bias here, but this I feel was a blatant betrayal of trust by men and women who were well aware of just what Norton's work had meant to the university as it sought to develop a reputation of serious academic and scientific endeavor and overcome its reputation of being "Suntan U."

Never one to linger long over setbacks, Ed Norton and his trusted director of development, Debra Durant, had already undertaken a five-year capital fundraising campaign of 23 million dollars to address the needs of the coming decade (there's that over-the-horizon radar again). With the funds they were able to finish the shell on the third floor in 1983, adding 27,000 square feet of badly needed space for glaucoma, with four faculty, and external, with six faculty members, that could not be contained in the existing clinical spaces, as well as a beautifully equipped pathology laboratory and eye bank for Vic Curtin.

What of the building vacated when BPEI moved across the street in to its new quarters? Did it lie fallow? Of course not. The reputation of the Institute by now was such that patients from all walks of life came to its doors for care. One was William L McKnight. His rise from being an office clerk at a small firm named Minnesota Mining & Manufacturing to the role of its long-term chairman and guiding genius as it became 3M is one of the true life Horatio Alger stories of a bygone generation. His company is a model of ethical American business at its innovative best.

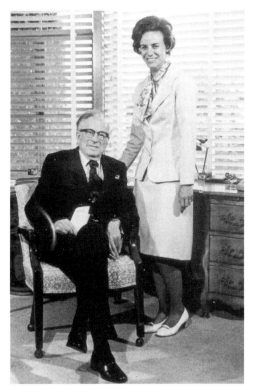

WILLIAM L. MC KNIGHT AND MARY LOU LEWIS

A sufferer from macular degeneration and a faithful patient of Mary Lou Lewis, as was his wife, he made a major gift that enabled the building originally planned to support eight floors to reach that height and by a clever remodeling of the face of the building to extend the floor space to reach a total space of 70,000 square feet. Needless to say the structure was renamed in his honor: the William L. McKnight Vision Research Institute. His success, as well as his company's, depended on research, and he intuitively recognized its value.

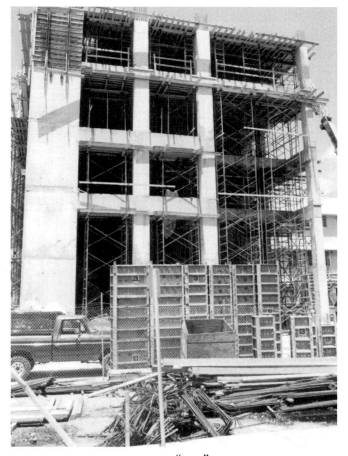

REMODELING OF THE "OLD" BPEI INTO THE MC KNIGHT VISION RESEARCH INSTITUTE

Ground was broken in 1986 and the remodeling completed in 1988, on schedule. As expected, there were two shell floors to allow for the future, by now a Norton trademark.

The McKnight Vision Research Institute houses some of the most productive laboratories in the nation dedicated to ophthalmology. Not least is Jean Marie Parel's Henri & Flore Lesieer ophthalmic biophysics laboratory, where vitrectomy instruments were developed and which now works in many diverse fields of clinically applied research, from lasers to biopolymers to tiny wide angle digital cameras. If one has a problem and it needs a fix badly, a visit to Jean Marie's office in his busy laboratory and workshop is likely to provide the first clear roadmap toward a solution.

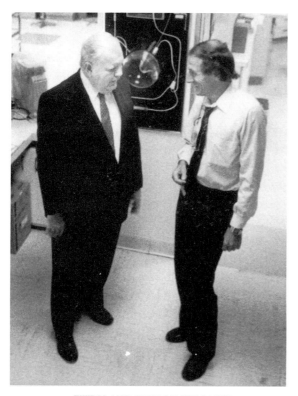

EWDN AND JEAN MARIE PAREL
IN THE BIOPHYSICS LABORATORY

The Norton era of building was slowly gliding to a soft landing. The last major project undertaken was the finishing of the shell space of the fourth floor of the BPEI/ABLEH. It provided clinic space for oculoplastics, neuro-ophthalmic and glaucoma services and the childrens clinic.

Additional office space was provided in the northwest corner of the building. For many years I had been complaining to my two fellow "Cornellies" how deprived I was of Florida sunshine, never having a window in any of the offices I had occupied in my years at BPEI. I was not loathe to point out to them how well they had provided for themselves with ample sunlight and view windows whereas I, sallow of complexion, labored in near Bastille-like darkness. It's an old Irish trait that loves to exaggerate woe just a bit when telling the tale to another Irishman. "Ah but God sees the truth and waits," goes the Gaelic saying.

Never ones to pass up a chance to turn a good trick on their junior Irish partner, they installed me in an office that had two of its four walls exclusively glass, floor to ceiling. They provided a lovely view and an artistic touch, but in the afternoons from April to November I had reason to regret that I ever opened my mouth. No heavy curtains or drapes could dim the implacable penetration of Helios' rays and the room's resemblance to an oven.

So in the best spirit I could muster I gritted my teeth and resolved never to whimper to my tormentors. And what did I get for my troubles? I was the one of the three Celts who developed the basal cells and actinic keratoses as my equally fair skinned Hibernians went scot-free. No pun intended!

The development office occupied the crook in the "L" of the building's footprint. Long deserved, this office was the dynamo that furnished the financial resources for the torrent of growth that had characterized the last era of Norton's work. Working there were Debra, almost a surrogate daughter, and Margaret, Cynthia, Janice, Frances, Eva, Julie and Wilma. This remarkable crew worked closely by Norton's side to fufill what he clearly saw as the needs of the BPEI and its hospital in the decades to come.

The picture, however, was becoming increasingly cloudy. Though the eye service was busier every year, revenues were flat. Which meant that everyone was working harder just to stay in the same place. A measure of success in its own right but hardly seen in that light in a world whose eyes are focused only on the bottom line.

Ed's work with the development office increasingly occupied his energies. Endowment was the very best hedge for the department and his faculty against the vagaries of the future in an uncertain world. Ed Norton knew better than anyone how uncertain that future world could be. The growth of the endowment was the best measure of how hard and successful his energies proved to be in this arena. It was said that one in four dollars raised on the medical campus was raised by BPEI. Palm Beach was a source of many of those dollars.

The trip to Miami became more and more arduous and demanding, at times even dangerous for patients, many of them elderly. Palm Beach was on Ed's drawing board for the future as his era drew to a close. The Bascom Palmer of the Palm Beaches was to offer chiefly the sevices that were in short supply in quantity and quality, one might say, in the area. These were primarily the services required by an elderly, retired population: retina-vitreous, glaucoma, anterior segment and, importantly, low vision.

By the time Anne Bates Leach and her friend, Celeste Sanford, had left this world for their eternal rest, Ed and Debra had developed a whole coterie of loyal friends and supporters. With the second generation of Palm Beach supporters, he set about finding the land, paying key visits to the city fathers, planning the first stages of what the new building would look like (remarkably like the BPEI in Miami), and finally assuaging the fears of the local ophthalmologists, just as he had done so well three decades before in Miami.

Space was rented for the advanced party of BPEI faculty in Palm Beach Gardens, a choice location for growth, and property across from the rental site evaluated for purchase. Having done this and on some level realizing that he could go no further, he stepped back, like the good craftsman he was, and looked at the work of his hand and was satisfied.

Ed Norton was ready to turn over the task of guiding the most dynamic eye department in the United States in the last half of the twentieth century to someone else.

CHAPTER 14

The Chief and His Faculty and Students

A PERSON WOULD NOT BE FAULTED IF HE OR SHE ACCOMPLISHED only a part of what Ed Norton did and nothing more. But the life we celebrate here gave back to the world a group of men and women trained in the finest traditions of medicine and the ethic that must accompany its practice.

At his retirement in 1991, he left a clinical faculty of over thirty academic ophthalmologists, many prominent leaders in their field. And a counter-cultural culture in which people who came to BPEI as faculty stayed on, in contrast to the "move out to move up" philosophy so widespread in academic circles. Possibly this was because the institution was free of the nasty little turf wars and petty ego battles that so drag down and encumber academic institutions all over the map.

It seems to go with the mindset of some academicians that if there are no battles to be fought, they will invent them. BPEI was from its inception miraculously free of that miasma. Each individual was valued for what he or she brought to the institution and each was seemingly effortlessly fitted into the jigsaw puzzle of a departmental grand design by the master builder of the faculty.

Asked by an incredulous group of academic chairs in ophthalmology at the Association of University Professors of Ophthalmology (AUPO) how he did it, he came up with a simple document—presented at the AUPO meeting in Naples, Florida, January 7, 1991—that says it all.

THE NORTON PRINCIPLES

1.   Integrity: the key essential, the element by which I recruit new faculty. Don't ask me how I do it, I don't know.

2.   Organization: have a plan.

3.   Predictable behavior: stay on track.

4.   Ability to prioritize: balance the attention necessary for the task.

5.   Credibility: back up what you say; be right.

6.   Flexibility: accept the eccentrics, don't try to change them; adapt to the needs of the individual faculty.

7.   Encouragement: promote individual development. "Be the best you can be."

8.   Development of key faculty: let them be the stars. Don't you try to be the brightest star in the universe.

9.   Ability to listen: give everyone a chance, you don't have to agree. "I appreciate your opinion about this, I just don't happen to agree."

10.   Capacity to delegate: issue responsibility and authority.

11.   Utilization of support personnel: get help in the subspecialty areas.

12.   Role as a caretaker: like a gardener: "Pick the plants, cultivate the flowers, watch the blooms."

13.   Implementation of decisions: back up what you plan; move ahead.

14.   Vision: see an outcome; plan for the future and orderly transition into new leadership.

15.   Loyalty to the institution: "Chairs and faculty may go, the department may change in strength, the institution is forever."

That was in itself a trademark of his faculty. He almost never had to weather the storms raised by the sometimes brilliant but deeply flawed character of academics elsewhere.

The language was spare, almost Lincolnesque. The insights into the wellsprings of nature, human nature, at least the human nature that seems to inhere in the breast of the academician was deep and broad. The emphasis was on not so much on intellectual talents, which are almost taken for granted, but on the more enduring and constant qualities best summed up by the word "character," necessary to live "an examined life," i.e., one worth living in the converse of Socrates' words of millennia ago: "He picked well, not flawlessly, but well."

That was in itself a trademark of his faculty. He almost never had to weather the storms raised by the sometimes brilliant but deeply flawed character of academics elsewhere.

During his tenure, he trained 187 residents and 373 fellows. Of this number, more than 125 are in fulltime academic positions and fifteen are or have been department chairs. Two have become deans. The most frequent refrain one hears from those fortunate enough to have spent all or part of their post-graduate education in ophthalmology at BPEI is, "It was the single best academic (or intellectual) experience of my life."

To permit each to have a voice here would prohibitively lengthen this book. Instead I have arbitrarily chosen from each of the decades, "Bascom Palmerites" to voice in their own words what the man and the institution meant to them. I believe that when taken together the words of these men and women will reflect a certain grandeur of the man and the institution with which all can agree.

The Fifties

His first fellow in retina, *Jose Berrocal and his wife, Pru,* parents of two ophthalmologists who themselves experienced part of their training at BPEI:

> *Ed and Mary Norton were the life of every party that*
> *we had as ophthalmologists. Mary Norton was the most*
> *charming ophthalmologist's wife of her generation.*

The Sixties

From the 1955 graduating class of the University of Miami, one of the most accomplished ophthalmologists ever trained at BPEI, in private practice in Pensacola, Florida, **Charley Clevenger**:

> *When I was an intern in 1956 at Jackson, Ophthal-*
> *mology was tucked away in a tiny corner of the outpatient*
> *clinic . . . when I returned four years later it had its own*
> *four-story building with more clinic space than Medicine*
> *and Surgery combined. At home in Birmingham (before I*
> *became a resident) Dr. Alston Callahan, helping me find a*
> *good residency program, called Dr. John Mc Lean in New*
> *York. He could not say enough good things about Dr. Norton.*
> *I was absolutely shocked to find that already there were*
> *thirty-three applicants for three places and one had already*
> *been given. All of us who were privileged to work with him*
> *already knew: he was one of the world's truly greatest men.*

A year behind Charley and an almost Gatsby-like figure of legend during his years in Miami, **Norm Ellerman**:

> *Norton was a master motivator of diverse talent and*
> *personalities, encouraging and supporting individuals to*
> *pursue their areas of interest. The clarity of thought, uncan-*
> *ny wisdom, pursuit of excellence, and long hours of hard*
> *work resulted in great accomplishments.*

One of the first graduates of BPEI to reach the academic heights of department chair and now happily ready to turn over that task to another, **Malcolm (Mike) Luxenberg** said:

Those were great years and I will always be grateful for the training I received and the outstanding people we had as mentors — not only as great teachers but as wonderful role models.

A true solid rock of the residency, **Ray Sever:**

I first met him when he was trying to teach students how to use a direct ophthalmoloscope. First he used the high diopter lens to look at the lids and conjunctiva. While doing this on a patient in the medical clinic I saw a funny vein that was only half filled with blood. I walked over to the eye clinic to ask Dr. Norton to look at this funny vein. He said it was a vein of Ascher.

I started my residency in 1964 as fluorescein angiography was beginning. I went next door to the medical library and looked up the absorption and emission spectra of fluorescein, went to the camera store on SW 8th Street and 12th Avenue and chose two filters. With the new filters we got a quantum jump in the quality of pictures. For the next two Friday afternoons Don Gass, Johnny Justice and myself reviewed the pictures for the week. It became obvious that this was going to be a good teaching session and fluorescein conference was established on Tuesday night.

The Chief's personality was exemplified by the way he ran grand rounds. Thursday morning was a time for the ophthalmologists in Miami to get together. They were welcomed and wanted. Clear questioning, logical train of thought and always the end product being good patient care characterized grand rounds and the Bascom Palmer.

Words cannot express the gratitude I feel for the three years I spent at Norton's Bascom Palmer and for the life I have spent enjoying the practice of ophthalmology.

Ray and Johnny Justice published in Lawton's first *Neuro-Ophthalmology Symposium* the very first description of the exciting barrier filter that took fluorescein angiography out of the dark, low-contrast age and into the high-contrast era in which it thrived as the diagnostic tool forever linked to the BPEI.

Joel Glaser, student of the Chief and JLS:

> *I was very fortunate because I first met Ed Norton in 1962 when I did a two month elective as a medical student with Lawton. Ed, Lawton and Nobby David enjoyed each other's company so much they would meet two or three times a week over at Pappas for lunch and exchange stories and cases and good bits of humor along with their presentations. . . .*

Percy Chee summed it up perhaps best another way:

> *My first impressions of the Chief have been lasting ones. Dr. Norton was a man of great humility, integrity, intelligence, with tremendous vision for innovations in Ophthalmology. In his presence, residents learned in an atmosphere that encouraged the thought process, even when one of us may have made some "dumb" statement to him. I can still recall haunting memories of the times I would report to him about something and he would simply say, "But Percy, don't you think . . ." bringing my total lack of judgment into focus in a most convincing and non-judgmental manner.*
>
> *Dr. Frank Bosquet was chief resident at New York Hospital when Ed was a resident. He shared this anecdote: "Dr. Sidney Werner, the famed Columbia thyroid expert was guest at grand rounds at NYH and announced to the group of doctors attending how fortunate they were to have in their midst a physician who had personally examined more than 100 thyroid eye disease patients, Dr. Edward Norton. Needless to say that came as a great shock to the chief resident.*
>
> *The Chief gave one the feeling of trust and made it clear that personal integrity was at the top of his list of characteristics he looked for in choosing his residents. Time and*

again, throughout the years, I witnessed those qualities displayed by him. I miss his wisdom, compassion, and encouragement.

Another academician who changed the face of modern retina-vitreous surgery, **Robert Machemer**:

> *It was amazing how he supported you morally and helped you be secure to go on, because you know how rapidly self-confidence can be destroyed when you are just beginning. Let me close on one aspect of his I admired, that he was not living for the moment . . . that he was always projecting into the future.*

Rounding out the decade, **Jim Cerasoli**, an ex-Marine and a Norton favorite as well:

> *The residents in my group were Dick Forster, George Dinter, Lee Duffner, and Larry Brenner. We worked very hard and enjoyed the entire experience. All this we credited to the Chief who we came to know as a special dynamic person. He brought out the best in us.*
>
> *I remember ophthalmology grand rounds each Thursday morning as his favorite forum for teaching. The residents were encouraged to present interesting patients. The Chief made it a tremendous teaching experience. Each year ended with Residents' Day. What a party! It was stressful but so rewarding—a wonderful culmination to each year. To me he was number one among all the greats in the field.*

The Seventies

Richard K. Forster, one of the early chief residents, longtime faculty member and interim chair of the Department during a turbulent transition for the institution:

I think we all felt that we could go to him about any-
thing, any problem, and I went to him with personal problems
and he took . . . it wasn't a superficial view of it. He sought
to console, to advise on a limited basis, but he listened, that
was the main thing, without judging. I think that was one
of the things I really loved about Ed Norton.

Joel Kramer, one of the BPEI's ambassadors to North Florida
where he is a senior ophthalmologist in Tallahasseee:

When I first walked into the Bascom Palmer Eye Insti-
tute thirty-five years ago, I knew nothing of ophthalmology
or of Dr. Edward Norton, other than the fact that he was
willing to take a chance on a young physician looking for a
meaningful way to experience a professional career.
*   Three years later I understood I had found not only a*
teacher, but a model whose clinical excellence and ability to
share that with those around him was matched only by the
gentle humanity with which he treated his patients, house
staff and faculty. I have to this day a picture of the Chief
behind my office desk. Sometimes, at the end of a long clinic
on a good day, I think I see him smile at my efforts.

John Shock, Chair of the Department of Ophthalmology at
Arkansas for 21 years and recently appointed interim Dean of the
College of Medicine, but declined to be a candidate. A West Point
graduate, John knows well when to duck. He has this to say
about the Chief:

Ed Norton's acceptance of me as a retinal fellow changed
my life. The key word was opportunity . . . to expand my hori-
zon and to learn about disease and life from him. Dr.
Norton was truly without peer in providing wisdom, fore-
sight and insight to those who worked closely with him.

Henry Clayman, former New York taxi driver and subject of Her Majesty, the Queen, after an eventful career as part of the intra-ocular lens revolution of the seventies and eighties, now gives days of volunteer time back to the residency that trained him and can always be counted on for a word or two on any subject addressed to us as "the colonists":

> *Dr. Norton's superior abilities and clinical acumen were quite apparent, notwithstanding his modesty. Less visible was his ability to communicate with both prince and pauper (plus all in between) and make them feel that they had his complete attention and total concern. I believe that this gift of his was pivotal in his recruitment and retainment of a distinguished faculty, superior housestaff, and the development of the best ophthalmology program in the world, with its culture of benevolent excellence. I miss him.*

Steve Charles, one of the finest and most innovative of BPEI's graduates in the field of retina-vitreous surgery, which, it might

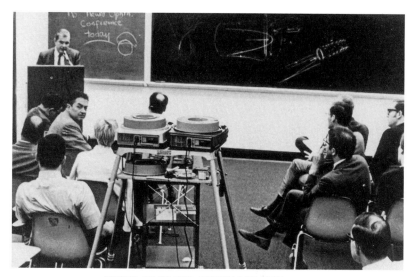

EWDN AT GRAND ROUNDS IN THE 1970s

be said with justification, was invented at BPEI, remembers a unique and poignant aspect of the Chief:

> *I worked in the OR as an orderly at night and got to know him when he spent three days at the bedside of a child who suffered a cardiac arrest during retinal detachment surgery. He adjusted her IV, mannitol, cooling blanket, read EEGs, did neurological exams and was incredibly concerned.*

Stanley Chang, now Edward Harkness Professor of Ophthalmology at Columbia and in the process of rebuilding that institution along the lines learned at BPEI says:

> *Edward Norton was a truly unique individual — a brilliant clinician and surgeon and an outstanding teacher. While not an active researcher, he recognized important areas of investigation and directed faculty and resources to develop them. His leadership guided talented faculty to make significant contributions that radically improved clinical care.*
>
> *As a teacher, Dr. Norton could make even the most routine patient turn into a learning adventure. His keen observational abilities would point out an interesting feature*

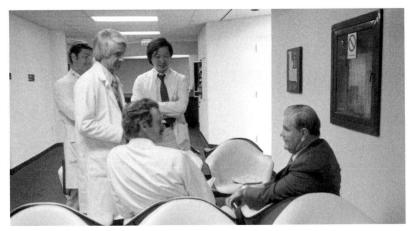

EWDN AND HIS FELLOWS: HARRY FLYNN, GARY ABRAMS, STANLEY CHANG

in almost every patient. The environment he and the faculty created at the Institute was intellectually and socially nonpareil. He made you part of a huge "family" and they continued to make you feel part of that family after completion of training. I am very grateful for the opportunity to grow in ophthalmology and personally from the Bascom Palmer experience.

Bill Stiles, our quintessential Chicago insider, lifelong admirer of the political finesse of both Richard J. Daley and Edward W.D. Norton who, in his words:

> *We always called him the Chief. Sometimes we called him Dr. Norton and the other professors called him Ed. As the past 30 years have slipped away, my understanding of Dr. Norton as Chief has greatly expanded beyond the title. "Chief" reflects so many shades and nuances of how Dr. Norton as leader led and how those who followed responded. Our understanding of the term tells not only who he was but how he changed our lives, our values, our ethics. You left believing that ophthalmology was just a wonderful specialty. He loved fluorescein conference and he much preferred having a number of faculty in attendance so the discussion would be lively. His examination of patients at grand rounds was detailed and invariably he saw something generally missed. He fostered open debate, and community ophthalmologists were partners.*
>
> *If the term "the Chief" means anything it means total commitment to excellence. When I think of Dr. Norton, the Chief stands for leadership of the highest order . . . not only leader but rabbi, priest, minister, confessor, tribal elder, mentor, story teller, mediator, visionary, doctor, surgeon, teacher, recruiter and most of all friend.*

One of that inimitable group of residents who had been college boys and girls of the sixties with Viet Nam, Woodstock and Mario

Savio, with all that portends, **Mike Barricks** speaks for his group:

> *Though very modest, the Chief was a brilliant clinician, teacher, administrator and builder. I always felt these achievements grew from the most remarkable skill of all, his incredible "people" skill. He brought out the best in us by humor, honesty, compassion, intellectual rigor, and emphasis on the highest ethical standards. He was always available to the residents.*

Lou Lobes, another of that group, adds:

> *The Chief naturally understood the intrinsic value of every human being. He treated clinic patients and professors all with the same respect. I have tried to carry this lesson throughout my life, and it has brought me comfort, friends from surprising places, and allowed me to truly love being a physician. I am grateful every day for that lesson.*

Rounding out the seventies, which from my vantage point was a vintage decade rich with bright, questioning, at times somewhat in a hurry for change, and a trifle rebellious group, but never beyond the ability of Victor to handle in his own remarkable way, **Ken Guerry,** who with Mike Barricks, Chad Sparrow and others produced probably the greatest Residents Day skit of all claims that

> *. . . in the mid-seventies Lawton Smith, without a doubt the most memorable teacher I ever encountered, quipped that he feared the ophthalmic community might join together in a lawsuit against the Chief on the grounds of what he called "Bone Up Practice." As usual, Lawton was onto something. All of us ran the risk of extreme frustration in trying to meet the exceptional standards Ed set for himself and, by his example, for the rest of us. In reality we took pride, all of us —*
> *resident, fellow, faculty member, community physician — in trying to elevate the level of our performance, and we felt*

flattered that he expected so much from us. There was a sense that you were privileged to be a part of what Ed was building, and also, I believe, a feeling that you just did not want to let him down. All of this was unspoken but palpable. The result, of course, made history.

The Eighties

Jerry Fisher rings in this decade for us. One of the excellent ophthalmologists that BPEI trained and who remain faithful in so many ways to their mother institution, Jerry practiced for years with Harry Horwich and the late Dave Kasner (names that will mean much to residents of the older vintage). Jerry's comment on "the Chief":

> *My first impressions of Dr. Norton came as an intervie-wee. He greeted me in a warm fashion and treated me as a fellow professional rather than as an exalted leader inter-viewing a lowly medical student applying for a residency position. He asked me for my opinions on serious problems potentially affecting the future of the residency. He paid attention to my responses and I came away from that meet-ing feeling that he actually was interested in my thoughts. In retrospect, I am sure that he was sizing me up in his own gentle way.*
>
> *What I subsequently came to understand was that the Chief was the consummate leader whose greatest strengths included his ability to pick the best people for the job and give them the tools to get that job done. He also had the wonderful leadership quality of being able to have people come to the very conclusions that he desired while allowing them to think that it was their idea all along. These qualities coupled with his unquestioned ethical principles made him the outstanding ophthalmic educator and leader of his era.*

Carl Wetzig, son of Paul, Ed's friend from NY Hospital days, who grew up with the Norton children, has this to say:

> *My path to ophthalmology possibly began at age four (1951) when my father and Dr. Norton outfitted us kids with operating room garb to wear trick or treating at 1303 York Avenue. The Norton/Wetzig families remained close over many years through gatherings, some even at major ophthalmological meetings where we were always included. I was able to witness the early development of the legend as it was happening.*
>
> *I vividly recall the Chief's enthusiasm for ophthalmology carrying over into vacation time — he had a half-hour conversation with my father about what he was doing with his first year residents while we were traveling an access road to the base of Mount Uncompaghre (14,000+ ft.) for a day's climb (1968). Dr. Norton didn't quite make the summit; every 10 minutes he took his pulse and announced what it was and added, "Pa-a-aul, when it reaches 150 I'm stopping." When the inspiration to pursue ophthalmology arrived the prospect of success in that career seemed much more intimidating due to my frame of reference for excellence: a keen awareness of the EWDN phenomenon.*
>
> *My future wife, Carol, and I enjoyed a personal relationship with the then recently widowed Dr. Norton. I learned the concept of a principle based approach to the specialty, for love of the process, devoid of encumbering economic concerns. In his closing remarks at his and Dr. Curtin's retirement dinner he reminded everyone of how proud he was to have trained all the individuals out there.*

Scotty Jaben, another of the many outstanding UM graduates that BPEI has attracted over the years commented:

> *There is never a single week that goes by that I do not think about my days at Bascom Palmer or my memories of Dr. Norton. The environment at the institute, the camaraderie*

and the professional experience that I encountered from my early days as a medical student and throughout my residency and fellowship training have never been matched nor taken for granted. The years at BP remain a very deep-seated source of pride and affection. Although there are many whose input made it so, the credit must start at the top.

We (the residents) would often compliment Dr. Norton about this and thank him for the opportunity to partake in the BP experience. His modest reply would always go something like this: "BP may be all of these things, but your growth and success is what you make of the opportunity . . . how you take advantage of the experience." I quote him often. I am constantly grateful for the chance to spend four busy and worthwhile years of my life at BP working with Dr. Norton and the entire staff.

Drew Levada, a member of the brightest or nearly so class ever to matriculate at the Institute and an admired and respected member of the Yale faculty expressed his thoughts quite well:

I had just finished another residency in internal medicine when I arrived in Miami. Dr. Norton came to see the residency group on the first day as we were being shepherded about by Dr. Michael Cobo, our chief resident. He personally gave me a Nikon 20-diopter indirect lens to use. It was a small gesture which immediately made him tower over my previous chief. This guy really cared about me. I still use that lens in my consult kit and think of him every time I use it.

The tone he set was that everyone was important. First came the patients, then came everyone else who was part of the team. No one could have a conflict that prevented them from devoting themselves to taking care of people. He didn't like people who did research or practiced medicine primarily to make a name for themselves rather than to make people better. That was the focal point of the Institute and it showed in everything.

Carlos Valdes Lora, aka Ca-a-hlos to certain faculty from northern climes, practices in South Mami:

> *I remember the Chief every time a patient thanks me for his or her surgery, for the miracle that is vision. Through great humility and patience, greatness found Dr. Norton; I suppose that is how he was able to put together so many wonderfully talented physicians that formed the most coveted faculty in the nation during our "Golden Years," a time he so aptly named. What a perfect opportunity that I will always treasure as a blessing, to have been able to grow in my profession at the Bascom Palmer.*

Karen Senikowich-Morgan, an attending at USC Doheny Eye Institute, remembers her days at BPEI:

> *Twenty years ago I arrived in Miami with high expectations. California had some good ophthalmology residency programs and Florida seemed a long way to go for an education. I wasn't the first female resident, but was the first from California. It didn't take long to realize that the entire Institute was the creation of one man. Every painting on the wall, each book in the library and the state-of-the-art equipment was there because of Dr. Norton. Most importantly, he had recruited an incredibly talented faculty.*
> *The Chief was the rare combination of a great leader and a very capable manager — and he loved Bascom. It was not a stepping stone to some higher position. Bascom was the position. The Institute was his life and its employees were his family. Kindness and generosity were Dr. Norton's hallmarks. As residents, he made us feel important. We were included in the fundraising balls and invited to his home for parties. As seniors, we all looked forward to dinner at the Academy with the Chief. His relationship with all of us was paternal. We sought his parental approval. After my first grand rounds presentation, Dr. Norton commended, "Isn't she something?*

That's my golden girl." Those words of praise meant so much to me.

Elaine Chuang, on the full-time faculty of the University of Washington and a gifted retina-vitreous surgeon says:

> *Prior to my Miami days, my ophthalmology mentors were already deep admirers of "the Chief." During my fellowship ('84) and then retina faculty days ('86–93), this was all borne out: the most honest and personable of men! Sharp clinical acumen, wise perspective on where medicine had been and was going . . . and always a kind look or word to everyone on the BPEI team. May I strive to model my "way of going" ever closer to that of EWDN!*
>
> *My most personal anecdote with the Chief pertains to my very straight hair and decision to get a perm for the first time as a fellow. An absolute disaster, to my eye! Despite the ghastly kinks, my inevitable next day at BPEI rolled around. We passed in the hall . . . the Chief did a double take, and then asked "What are you doing with your hair?" Recognizing my discomfort, after a pause he gently added, "Change is good."*

Allan Slomovic, one of the nicest persons ever to grace our institution. Allan is currently a faculty member at University of Toronto:

> *Dr. Norton was a unique individual who helped me through a difficult time in my professional career. I remember him as a remarkable listener who always made you feel that he had your best interests at heart and that you had his support. What I remember most about Dr. Norton was his compassionate manner and his comforting words and advice. It is said that "every dark cloud has its silver lining"; for me the silver lining was that I had the privilege of getting to know this remarkable individual who in many ways has served as a role model for me.*

Steve Russell, another of BPEI's donations to academia and a more recent visitor to Residents Day had this to say:

> *Each year I have an increased appreciation for Dr. Norton and his contributions. One day as a second year resident, I accompanied him during his entire clinic day at Bascom Palmer. For me, the prospect of observing the attending for a day raised the specter of boredom. But I had observed Dr. Norton for years as a department chairman, moderator of grand rounds, and suspected that his personal charisma and optimism would make the time worthwhile. That day remains a highlight of my career as I watched Dr. Norton deftly examine, educate, and manage the most demanding group of patients I have seen. He diagnosed one high maintenance patient with Irvine-Gass syndrome. Another he simply reassured. His chairside manner was astounding.*
>
> *He represents so many ideals. He was a chairman who cared more about the development and progression of his faculty, fellows and residents than for himself. He was a researcher who understood and cared most for the human nature of his patients. For me he is a personal hero.*

Scott Snead, in practice with Jack Sipperly in the wild "free market" of Arizona ophthalmology; both men bring credit to the program where they trained. Scott says:

> *Dr. Norton will live on in my mind as a man of many admirable qualities. He was an astute and charismatic chairman, stressing the importance of choosing residents who could work together in a productive and cooperative manner. He was a caring and attentive educator who enjoyed taking the residents out to dinner with visiting professors and during Academy meetings. He treated me and the other residents with the same respect and kindness that he demonstrated towards the faculty, patients and clinic staff. He always*

stressed that quality patient care was the primary duty of the ophthalmologist.

I am grateful to have had the opportunity to serve as a resident under his stewardship of Bascom Palmer and shall always remember the warmth not only of his smile but of his character.

Judy Hustead settled the tiresome controversy between ophthalmology and optometry by marrying an optometrist, Paul Marvin, OD, whom she met at BPEI and lives happily ever after. She recalls Ed Norton:

During my residency years from 1985–1988, I had little opportunity to work directly with Dr. Norton. There was no question, however, that he set the standard for absolute professional integrity and unwavering commitment to patient care in the present and the future.

Her husband, **Paul Marvin**:

I was very fortunate to work in Dr. Norton's clinic. I will always remember him sitting at the slit lamp with his elbow on the table. He was listening to his patient. He knew each patient as an individual and understood their need to talk and to have their doctor listen.

Deanna Wilson, one of our chief residents and reputed to be (with George Hilton, another BPEI alum) the best retina surgeon in the Bay Area. Deanna, a gentle Iowa farm girl remembers:

. . . the first time I met him and the ease of which I sat with him over a cup of coffee, and he the wise, quietly critical, bear of a man who I had only heard about. I know now why I felt so comfortable. He was so human in the way he cared about his hospital, his doctors and his patients. He

was a man of integrity that you knew would give you a fair shake. I worked for Dr. Norton for four very good years. He commanded my absolute respect. I consider him and Bascom Palmer to be a turning point for me — a launching pad.

I remember walking down the hallway with him having a discussion about women and the chief residency. He picked my brain on what I thought and that it broke with their tradition, and then allowed me that great privilege a few days later. The last time I saw him was in Mill Valley, California with his daughter and family at a restaurant. I had my first son with me! And he was still the supportive wonderfully insightful man who I will remember forever as "family" in so many ways.

The Nineties

Steve Fransen, another of those incredibly bright Don Gass fellows who came to study at the foot of the master and added so much to the intellectual life of the Institute during their time here:

In the summer of 1989 I joined a renaissance known as Bascom Palmer Eye Institute. Don Gass was my greatest source of inspiration that year, his towering powers of observation and reason exceeded only by his humility and warmth. Although Dr. Gass was friends with everyone, it became apparent he shared a special bond with Ed Norton. Their relationship first benefitted me directly when Dr. Gass told me, "Ed just approved" our purchase of a slide scanner to pursue my interest in digital retinal imaging. In 1989 digital retinal imaging was far from the beaten path but that didn't dampen their enthusiasm. I still hear the excitement in Dr. Norton's voice, encouraging me to forge ahead with my ideas despite what must have seemed like incomprehensible rambling on my part about spatial resolution, pixel depth, and other nuances of digital imaging. Later that year, Dr.

Norton handed me a set of stereo color slides; the pride in his voice was palpable as I was able to correctly differentiate the case as rubella retinopathy. His personal commitment to my education remains etched in my mind more than a decade later.

Ed Norton and Don Gass gave us their gifts of knowledge, humility, respect and kindness. I hope we will steward these gifts and pass them along to those who follow. During a conversation with Don Gass several years ago, he concluded by simply saying, "I sure miss Ed."

Pat Rubsamen, a former faculty member now in private practice in Broward, sees the institution from both perspectives:

When one reflects on what Edward W.D. Norton meant to the people around him, they might think of academics pursued, a premier eye hospital constructed or a world-class eye department and training institution created, and certainly all of those things would be true. But when I think of Ed Norton I think of people. I think of the personal impact this great man had on so many lives. He certainly touched my life and altered it in a way for which I will always be thankful.

Dr. Norton taught me two of the most important lessons that I learned in my medical training. First, treat patients as you would want them to treat you. And second, enjoy the most important aspect of patient care, the opportunity to meet so many special people under special circumstances. When I once asked Dr. Norton what he valued most in his career, he said, "It was the opportunity to meet and know so many interesting people." The Chief is gone but certainly not forgotten.

Barb Blodi, resident and then fellow, now at the University of Wisconsin, Madison, one member of the only brother-sister team of BPEI residents, had this to say:

One of the indelible memories I have of Dr. Norton was during a meeting of the retinal surgeons on Wednesday mornings in the BPEI inpatient floor lounge. One of the surgical fellows was describing a long, complicated vitrectomy where things had gone badly for the surgeon, and the outcome for the patient was certain blindness. The fellow, when he was asked how often he would see the patient in follow-up, mumbled in response, "as little as possible." Dr. Norton jumped into the conversation at that point. In a stern but fatherly way he recommended instead that surgeons who had complications during their surgery should see their post-operative patients first thing in the morning every day (seven days a week) until the patient asks if he or she can come on a less frequent basis. Patients need to be told the nature of the complications and have as much time as they require with their surgeon. This approach, Dr. Norton explained, allows patients to better understand their condition and rebuilds trust and confidence between doctor and patient. Dr. Norton clearly loved seeing patients and it had a tremendously positive influence on me.

With these words of the residents and fellows who were representative of the many others selected during Ed Norton's watch, we close this chapter on his life. Sure, he participated in choosing the residents for several years after he resigned as chair. Sure, he was a presence about the Institute. But he was no longer in that comfortable, disarrayed office on the first floor of the McKnight, having moved to a small office on the sixth floor. He no longer ran grand rounds, having ceased that task in 1991. EWDN had finished the work he had come to do and turned the job over to others. But surely, we told ourselves, he would still be there for us if we needed him. And so he was. But for how little time!

CHAPTER 15

Ed Norton and His Community

THE MIAMI COMMUNITY SOON REALIZED THE WORTH OF THE MAN who quietly came into their midst in 1958. They responded with universal appreciation of his efforts to teach by example and to lead by gentle persuasion.

The phrase "town-gown," often used as shorthand to describe tension and animosity between these communities, found no place in the world he created around his department. Patients were seen by the faculty only on referral from an ophthalmologist seeking the help of the subspecialist at BPEI. And always referred back to the physician who had sent the patient. The bond of trust was ever there and rather than seeing the Institute as a threat, the community quickly recognized as a wonderful resource.

Grand rounds was the academic high point of the week for the faculty, the residents and fellows, and the private ophthalmologists. Patients instinctively knew that by being seen at grand rounds they were important to their doctor and the other physicians in attendence. (Unfortunately, the wonderful custom that Ed Norton began of bringing in coffee and danish and bagels could not continue forever. If for no other reason than the appetities of the residents and the number of private ophthalmologists who flocked to grand rounds!)

There was a spirit of learning, of careful inquiry that started with a thorough examination of the patient, and no one was more careful than the moderator himself. There was spirited argument by strongly opinionated practitioners presided over with tolerance and good humor by a master.

Ralph Kirsch, MD, perhaps his closest friend, supporter and colleague from the community, spoke of his long and cherished years with Ed (recorded at his home on April 10, 1998): "Let's begin at the beginning . . . John McKenna who was temporary head of Ophthalmology told me he had met Ed Norton and was very much impressed with him . . . I had in my mind a picture of this great big fellow, broad shouldered, athletic, powerful, with a brain of the same magnitude.

So I went to the OR at Jackson at 7:15 AM where he was operating and here comes somebody wearing blue scrubs and I said, 'would you be Ed Norton?' And he said 'yes' and I introduced myself. Well, instead of a great big tall fellow he was kind of a short, stocky man who walked with a slight bosun's rolling walk, but he had a face that was as Irish as Paddy's pig, kind, radiating warmth and honesty, his eyes looked at you and from that first minute I knew here was a guy I was really going to like. And that's the way it was throughout our time together—1958 to 1994.

"Everybody loved Ed Norton, from faculty colleagues to other departments' faculty to nurses, technicians, janitors and so on; they loved him and respected him. And grand rounds, that was something we had never known before . . . we would have live patients so everybody could examine them in the side rooms . . . and then the fun would begin . . . and there was very serious ophthalmology at a level we had never had before, and we had humor because Ed had a sense of humor that was glorious, and we all developed in the spirit our own senses of humor, so we had a great time besides learning a lot.

"Through all this Ed Norton grew and we all grew. And the only thing that worried me about him was when I saw him reach over at a scuttlebutt (naval slang for drinking fountain) and take a mouthful of aspirin, which he did frequently (he kept a giant jar in his desk). I didn't know what his pain was but this was a man in pain. Of course I would never have inquired as to the nature of it."

Ralph left us in 2000. A great loss to the Miami Community.

I'll close this chapter with one more comment from a long-time supporter of Ed's, Bob Welsh. (I do not mean in any way to slight the rest of the Miami community who, I'm quite sure, with individual variation would echo the sentiments of these two men.)

Bob Welsh speaks as he always did from the hip, and from the heart: "Previous to Dr. Norton's arrival our success rate for aphakic retinal detachment was ten percent. When Dr. Norton operated it was ninety-five percent. His residents began to get excellent results too. Dr. Ed Norton became a marvelous fundraiser for the Bascom Palmer Eye Institute. He raised more than $40 million, much more. I am convinced that it should be named the "Ed Norton Eye Institute.""

CHAPTER 16

L'Envoi

BEFORE WE FINISH, LET US SUMMARIZE WHAT ED NORTON AC-
complished in his thirty-four years at the helm in Miami. At the
very start he had two small offices and an examining room in the
old east wing of Jackson Hospital. His first efforts (in the early sixties) at changing the environment around him, little noticed or
long remembered by many, was to take his and Victor Curtin's
excess earnings, and air condition, clean, paint and upgrade the
creature comforts of the wards of the east wing where the Negroes
(as they were called) were forced by Jim Crow, still alive and well
in South Florida, to be hospitalized.

He could not change the culture so he did not waste the effort
and goodwill trying. But he made the sentinel gesture on behalf of
what was right several years after Brown versus the Board of Education and almost a decade before the Voting Rights Act of 1965.

Although planning and fundraising for the Bascom Palmer (the
"old," that is) was well under way before he came, his personal
intervention with Claude Hemphill was crucial to its successful
construction and showed his talent for "over the horizon" thinking
and planning with its fourth floor as a shell and a foundation to
support eight floors its final structure, once again with an eighth
shell floor for the future.

Thus was added a total of more than 300,000 square feet of
office and laboratory space to the university, and to the medical
school that held title to all the buildings (without contributing a
nickel to the costs of their construction). So strongly did he believe
in the symbiosis of a vibrant, growing department in an academic
home, having witnessed the somewhat ambiguous and tenuous
existence of Manhattan Eye and Ear as a model to avoid at all

January 11, 1963

Dr. Victor T. Curtin
1638 N. W. 10th Avenue
Miami 36, Florida

Dear Vic,

I am writing to thank you, in a more formal way, for your many contributions to the development of the Department of Ophthalmology, particularly during the past year.

I realize that many chores have fallen to you because of my involvement in administrative duties; you have accepted these with a minimum of upset. Specifically, the responsibility of the student teaching program, the "red tape" of the Eye Bank, the supervision of resident detachment surgery, interviewing residents, and the numerous private patients who have required your care.

In addition to these efforts, the monies you have spent in helping to equip the building as well as those recently deposited in the extra-mural account of the Department are deeply appreciated. I well realize the sacrifices you have had to make to earn these funds. I wish I could promise that the coming year will be easier - I can only hope it will be.

While I receive much credit for the development of the Department, I am well aware of your contributions and know better than anyone else how much the School is indebted to you. Each new staff member has an easier road because of those of us who have gone before.

Again, thank you.

Sincerely,

Edward W. D. Norton, M. D.

EWDN/gts

LETTER TO VTC FROM EWDN, 1963

costs, that I don't think he could believe otherwise.

His major contribution, however, came with the building that was to house the Bascom Palmer Eye Institute/Anne Bates Leach Eye Hospital. It encompassed within its walls 300,000 square feet of space. But more, much more: it provided a model for the very latest in in- and outpatient care in the United States of the seventies. And as the culture of health care changed under the grinding force of governmental and "for profit" medical care, he was able to remake it as an outpatient surgical center well ahead of the crowd of the anomalous, free standing, unregulated, indeed unobserved and often poorly financed and managed creatures of the mass market medicine that later came into being.

He thus was able to provide a decent model of how to do it right from the outset, a model that was largely ignored by the predators who had invaded, nay had been invited in by the confused medical profession that had lost, in this member's view at least, its vision of what its role was and is in a civilized society.

In summary, this is the material legacy that the humble builder left. He gave of his skill and talents freely to the institution that gave him a small place in which to do it. He asked for nothing except opportunity from them and got nothing else from them. It was all he ever needed. If one does nothing but count these material blessings left behind, he is without doubt the single greatest benefactor in the history of the University of Miami.

His name appears only inside the portals of the library he loved, the Mary and Edward Norton Library. He would have wanted it that way.

There is one more issue that deserves mention. For the last decade of his chairmanship he had, in effect, chosen his successor. Ed Norton would never leave a choice so important as this to the sometimes foolish whims of an academic search committee. Although he did not in any way attempt to bypass that institution, he carefully groomed and prepared his successor, John G. Clarkson.

We had all known John since his days as a medical student, when he worked with Don Gass on a summer project involving the angioid streaks in the retina in Paget's disease of bone. As a resident after military service, and chief resident after a fellowship at Johns Hopkins Wilmer Institute, he seemed to all the man for the job.

Ed saw to it that John was exposed to the wider world of the leaders of American and International Ophthalmology as well as the critical elements of management of a sixty million dollar a year business in ABLEH. It was a process we all watched with anticipation, admiration and delight. A job well done with the thoroughness so characteristic of Norton. We all wished John's tenure to be successful, as much for Ed's sake as his own. And so on June 1, 1991, Ed turned over the reins to John.

But it was not to be as Ed and John may have wished. For whatever reason, John felt more and more called to meet the needs of a sorely troubled and debt-ridden medical school, his alma mater, and began to take a more and more active role in its affairs instead of the department's.

Ed was aware of the shift—he could not avoid it, as shrewd an observer as he was—though he never spoke a word of disappointment to anyone. John Clarkson resigned the Edward W.D. Norton chair in 1996 to become Vice President for Medical Affairs and Dean of the University of Miami School of Medicine, a post he holds to this day.

As for Ed, he carried on as he always had, without a murmur. In his last days he was a presence somewhat in the shadows. Came to rounds and offered his opinion if asked, always wisely and judiciously given. Though he had retired he was always there for us. But his office was on the fifth floor of the old BPEI, not easy to get to and the door was not always open as it had been for us in the past.

The last years of his life, as described by Patty Norton Laird, his daughter and next door neighbor, were almost idyllic for him.

On coming home from a not-too-taxing day, he liked nothing better than to float in the water of his pool, warmed by the subtropical Miami sun, talking to his daughters and friends on the cordless phone. (Remember, this was a man who, in his lifetime, experienced the crank handle telephone, for sure the party line with the local operator who knew everybody's business, and even the days during the Great Depression when not every home had a phone.) Ed Norton was always one to appreciate life's small details that made it more liveable.

We all noted a wonderful change in the man. He had time. Time to have a conversation with whomever he met, time to linger over small delights — a picture, a phrase from a book. He always seemed in the past to have time for everyone else; now it seemed he had time for himself!

One could have a conversation with him about the fate of the hapless Bosox, about to blow another pennant to the Yankees. Even a conversation about the fortunes of the Notre Dame Fighting Irish football team without it leading to any true solution as, in fact, sports conversations are never meant to, are they? We all rejoiced for him and shared what we could of our delight at his release from the care of the chairmanship.

In 1985 he and Bruce Spivey took a trip to China as "the Odd Couple" in a group of Academy friends: Brad and Ruth Straatsma, Marshall and Angeline Parks, Stan and Dottie Truhlsen, Tom and June Hutchinson, and Tom and Marylou Kearns.

And in a completely different mode, Ed Norton as hard bargainer for a carved bowl, completed its purchase at close to his (and the seller's) price. It now graces the Mary and Edward Norton Library.

During those final years his grandchildren, numbering now twelve, were a great source of joy to him. Each was treasured as a unique individual. Each brought a part of the Norton legacy to him in physical form. Some of the older ones called him "Grandpere"

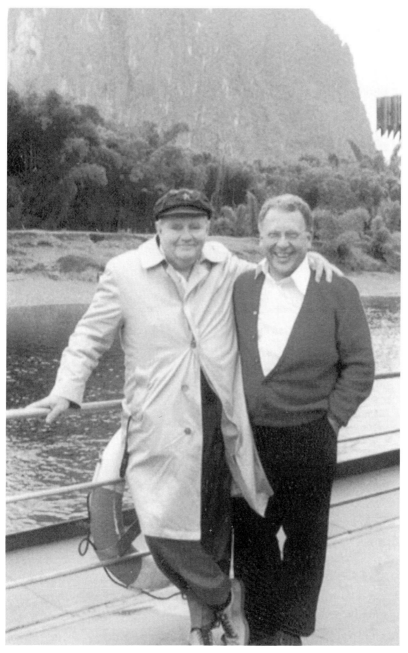

ED NORTON AND BRUCE SPIVEY ON THE YANGTZE RIVER

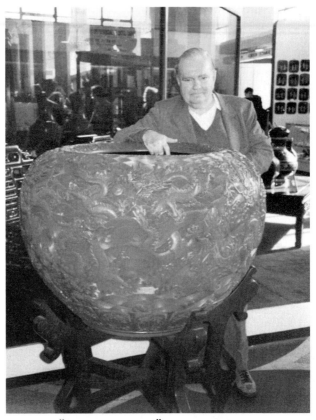

THE "HARD BARGAINER" WITH HIS PURCHASE,
THE CARVED BOWL

to distinguish him somehow from an ordinary grandpa. The younger enjoyed their grandfather for what grandfathers do best: they have time and an ear to listen and a hug to give.

Michael, his oldest grandson recalls wistfully: "At age 16 I worked for Jean Marie Parel at Bascom Palmer. That summer I got pretty close to my grandfather since we were living together, just the two of us, and driving to and from work together. I really enjoyed living with Grandpere and I remember wishing I could just stay there. I think he enjoyed it too, even though I think he was not completely at ease being thrust into the role of a single dad to a teenager."

Jennifer, his oldest granddaughter, recalls, "Traveling with Grandpere was so different from traveling with my own family. We stayed in fancy hotels, had cars take us around, and always had an evening cocktail. I never thought of Grandpere as old because he continued to work; he worked hard on his presentations. It's how I usually think of him now: with his briefcase walking away from me."

Ed's sister Polly Boyle and her husband managed, when each winter the snow flew in the northeast, to stay with him in the big, now almost empty house on Bayshore. Polly fussed over him, doted on him, chided and probably nagged him as sisters have done from time immemorial. He loved the attention!

We all carry with us a picture of him that seems somehow to

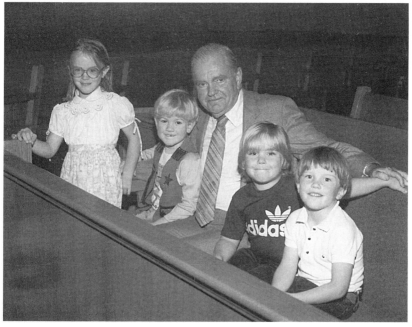

EWDN AND HIS GRANDCHILDREN

capture how we, in our frailty, would remember him best.

His daughter Patti recounts: "My dad decided to learn to sail in the years after Mom died. He took sailing classes at Ponce de Leon middle school in the evening adult education program. He fully acquainted himself with all things nautical through this class and books before asking Jack and Mary Lou Lewis to give him hands-on instructions.

"Shortly thereafter he purchased a 27-foot Catalina that he loved to sail with family and friends. He named it the 'Consultation' so his secretary Yvonne could tell people he was on consultation when they called and he wasn't in." (The picture of Ed Norton at play and enjoying to the hilt was taken by Ed Alfonso on an outing on the boat.)

Somehow he had been the helmsman to so many of our lives

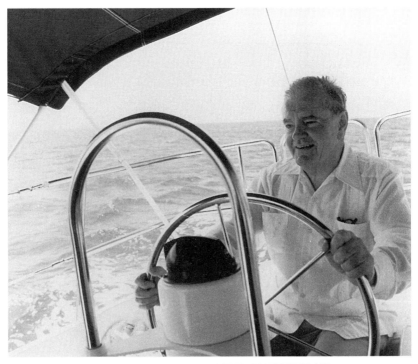

EWDN ON HIS SAILBOAT, THE CONSULTATION

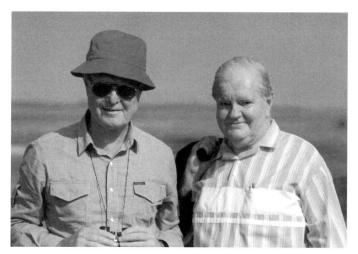

ED NORTON AND PAUL WETZIG IN COLORADO

for so long, it seemed quite natural to see him enjoy taking the helm of his own boat.

A reunion of the Norton and Wetzig families in Colorado in 1990 brought together for the last time the two friends, now both having accomplished much in their lives, each in his own sphere, each treasuring the times they shared together and the shared time of the two families for over four decades.

We were all dimly aware that his health in those last years was not as robust as it once seemed. But nothing that was not treatable. After all, he was of that tough Boston Irish stock who in so many ways resembled Jimmy Cagney, the actor-singer-dancer, born of that tough Hell's Kitchen Irish stock, was he not? Little did we realize how soon that familiar sight of him, his rolling bosun's gait, carrying his brown briefcase, with a slight, shy smile of recognition on his face as he approached, would soon be gone.

On Sunday morning, July 24, 1994, Edward Walter Dillon

Norton left us, quietly in his sleep. A man who more than any I know exemplified by his works the truth of Ignatious of Loyola's words that character is the will and action. A man whose works continue to this day, as Carlyle said, "Nothing that was worthy in the past departs; no truth or goodness realized by this man ever dies or can die, but is still here, and recognized or not, lives and works through endless changes."

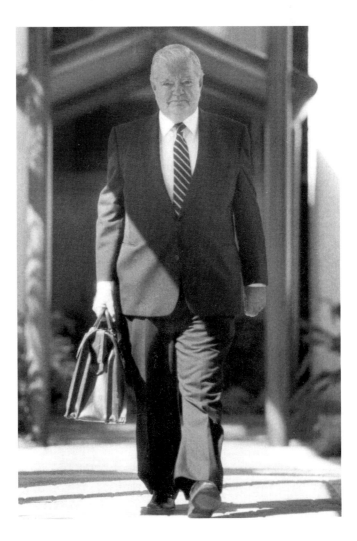

Acknowledgements

Many, many people can claim partial paternity or maternity of this work, if such a state can exist. My hope is that I do not overlook the contribution of any of them to its birth. If I do it is only because I am having what is known today in the delicacy of our politically correct language as a "senior moment." I can only hope that memory kicks in sometime before the manuscript reaches the printed page and I can add them to the list.

I want to acknowledge the contribution of Edward and Mary Norton's children and grandchildren, and Ed's sister, Mary Elizabeth (Polly) Norton Boyle. Without their generous and gentle help and guidance this book would be full of egregious error. Their love and devotion to Ed and Mary, very individual in each person, shines throughout the work. Each has my admiration, respect and love:

Carol Ann Norton Rogers – San Francisco, California
Brian Norton – Tallahassee, Florida
Mary Beth Norton Durant – Washington, DC
Kevin Norton – Tallahassee, Florida
Patti Norton Laird – Miami, Florida
Aunt Polly Norton Boyle – Naples, Florida
Michael John Norton – Washington, DC
Jennifer Rogers – San Francisco, California

I would also like to acknowledge the help of five very special people. Vic Curtin, my conscience as he was Ed's, has guided me factually, softened my Irish temper, and given me an overall feeling for the early building of BPEI. Next, my dear Reva Hurtes, librarian *extraordinaire*. She gave me full access to the Mary and Edward Norton Library and its facilities. And Doris Silver, the archivist who made available to me the fruits of her dedicated labors in compiling and cataloguing the many artifacts of Ed's life. Without that backbone this work would have been impossible. Jean Newland for suggesting the title as I wandered around aimlessly with hundreds that didn't fit while the one was staring me right in the face. And Rick Stratton, the maestro of the art of the computer, and I say that advisedly, for at his level it is an art. From scanning to cropping to cleaning—he can do it all. The cover design is largely his.

Deepest thanks for the patience, perseverance, tolerance and good humor of my editor and publisher, Lorna Rubin of Triad Publishing, Gainesville, Florida. She, too, became, as I was, obsessed with seeing this work through to its end, in spite of few short weeks allotted for her part in the project. Without her efforts on its behalf, I'm not sure it would have gotten done.

My dear wife Roseanne encouraged me to "stop talking and get going," as she has done so often in our life together.

My secretary of thirty years, Mary Jeanne Williams, organized my work and saw to two thousand details necessary to get it done.

I want to acknowledge all those who participated with me by granting me an interview or furnishing me with tape or fax or e-mail. Their insights have contributed immensely to the dimensions of Ed Norton's life and work that I surely would have overlooked without them. I am in debt to all, as all added to the picture of "the Chief."

Douglass Anderson
Patsy Carnahan
John Clarkson
Fred Cowell
Victor Curtin
Noble David
Edward Dunlap
Bernard Fogle
Edward Foote

Richard Forster
J. Donald and MargAnn Gass
Duco Hamasaki
Thomas Hedges
Ditte Hess
Irene Holmes
Reva Hurtes
Peter Jefferson
Yvonne Karrenberg
Ralph Kirsch
Gaby Kressly
Mary Lou Lewis
Jean Newland
Guy O'Grady
Marshall Parks
Fritz and Janet Schroeder
Thorne Shipley
J. Lawton Smith
William Spencer
Bruce Spivey
Henry K. Stanford
Robert Welsh
Paul Wetzig

Where it shines through in all its brilliance the credit belongs to my collaborators. Where it is foggy and seems to lose its way the responsibility is mine. This book celebrates the life of a very human man. He would understand.

And finally, thanks to those ex-residents and fellows whose comments are the substance of Chapter 14:

Jose Berrocal – San Juan, Puerto Rico
Charles Clevenger – Pensacola, Florida

Norman Ellerman – Palm Springs, California

Malcolm Luxenberg – Augusta, Georgia

Ray Sever – Temple Terrace, Florida

Percy Chee – Honolulu, Hawaii

Robert Machemer – Durham, North Carolina

James Cerasoli – Littleton, Colorado

Richard Forster – Miami, Florida

Joel Kramer – Tallahassee, Florida

John Shock – Little Rock, Arkansas

Henry Clayman – Miami, Florida

Steve Charles – Memphis, Tennessee

William Stiles – Northbrook, Illinois

Michael Barricks – Piedmont, California

Louis Lobes – Pittsburgh, Pennsylvania

R. Kenyon Guerry – Richmond, Virginia

Stanley Chang – New York, New York

Jerome Fisher – Miami, Florida

Carl Wetzig – Colorado Springs, Colorado

Scott Jaben – Charlotte, North Carolina

Andrew Levada – Waterbury, Connecticut

Carlos Valdes Lora – Miami, Florida

Karen Senikowich-Morgan – Pasadena, California

Elaine Chuang – Seattle, Washington

Annan Slomovic – Toronto, Canada

Steven Russell – Iowa City, Iowa

Scott Snead – Phoenix, Arizona

Judy Husted – Charlotte, North Carolina

Paul Marvin – Charlotte, North Carolina

Deanna Wilson – San Raphael, California

Steve Fransen – Oklahoma City, Oklahoma

Patrick Rubsamen – Fort Lauderdale, Florida

Barbara Blodi – Madison, Wisconsin